The Digestive System in the Era of COVID-19

The Digestive System in the Era of COVID-19

Editors

Daniel Paramythiotis
Eleni Karlafti

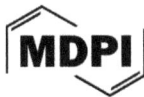 Basel • Beijing • Wuhan • Barcelona • Belgrade • Novi Sad • Cluj • Manchester

Editors
Daniel Paramythiotis
Aristotle University of Thessaloniki
Thessaloniki
Greece

Eleni Karlafti
Aristotle University of Thessaloniki
Thessaloniki
Greece

Editorial Office
MDPI
St. Alban-Anlage 66
4052 Basel, Switzerland

This is a reprint of articles from the Special Issue published online in the open access journal *Medicina* (ISSN 1648-9144) (available at: https://www.mdpi.com/journal/medicina/special_issues/7FH5N7FN9B).

For citation purposes, cite each article independently as indicated on the article page online and as indicated below:

Lastname, A.A.; Lastname, B.B. Article Title. *Journal Name* **Year**, *Volume Number*, Page Range.

ISBN 978-3-7258-0571-6 (Hbk)
ISBN 978-3-7258-0572-3 (PDF)
doi.org/10.3390/books978-3-7258-0572-3

© 2024 by the authors. Articles in this book are Open Access and distributed under the Creative Commons Attribution (CC BY) license. The book as a whole is distributed by MDPI under the terms and conditions of the Creative Commons Attribution-NonCommercial-NoDerivs (CC BY-NC-ND) license.

Contents

About the Editors vii

Preface ix

Bogdan Mihnea Ciuntu, Gheorghe G. Balan, Mihaela Buna-Arvinte, Irina Mihaela Abdulan, Adelina Papancea, Ștefan Lucian Toma, et al.
Clostridium difficile Infections in an Emergency Surgical Unit from North-East Romania
Reprinted from: *Medicina* 2023, 59, 830, doi:10.3390/medicina59050830 1

Kadir Gisi, Sukru Gungor, Murat Ispiroglu and Bulent Kantarceken
Could an Increased Percentage of Immature Granulocytes Accompanying Dyspepsia Predict COVID-19?
Reprinted from: *Medicina* 2022, 58, 1460, doi:10.3390/medicina58101460 10

Petros Bangeas, Nikolaos Konstantinidis, Tania Chrisopoulou, Despoina Karatzia, Alexandros Giakoustidis and Vasileios N. Papadopoulos
Small Bowel Diverticulosis and COVID-19: Awareness Is the Key: A Case Series and Review of the Literature
Reprinted from: *Medicina* 2024, 60, 229, doi:10.3390/medicina60020229 19

Xanthippi Mavropoulou, Elisavet Psoma, Angeliki Papachristodoulou, Nikoletta Pyrrou, Ekaterini Spanou, Maria Alexandratou, et al.
Gastrointestinal Imaging Findings in the Era of COVID-19: A Pictorial Review
Reprinted from: *Medicina* 2023, 59, 1332, doi:10.3390/medicina59071332 32

Sandica Bucurica, Florentina Ionita Radu, Ana Bucurica, Calin Socol, Ioana Prodan, Ioana Tudor, et al.
Risk of New-Onset Liver Injuries Due to COVID-19 in Preexisting Hepatic Conditions—Review of the Literature
Reprinted from: *Medicina* 2023, 59, 62, doi:10.3390/medicina59010062 46

Eleni Karlafti, Daniel Paramythiotis, Konstantina Pantazi, Vasiliki Epameinondas Georgakopoulou, Georgia Kaiafa, Petros Papalexis, et al.
Drug-Induced Liver Injury in Hospitalized Patients during SARS-CoV-2 Infection
Reprinted from: *Medicina* 2022, 58, 1848, doi:10.3390/medicina58121848 61

Georgios Geropoulos, Stavros Moschonas, Georgios Fanariotis, Aggeliki Koltsida, Nikolaos Madouros, Evgenia Koumadoraki, et al.
Anastomotic Leak and Perioperative Outcomes of Esophagectomy for Esophageal Cancer during the COVID-19 Pandemic: A Systematic Review and Meta-Analysis
Reprinted from: *Medicina* 2024, 60, 31, doi:10.3390/medicina60010031 75

Eleni Karlafti, Dimitrios Tsavdaris, Evangelia Kotzakioulafi, Adonis A. Protopapas, Georgia Kaiafa, Smaro Netta, et al.
The Prevalence of Gastrointestinal Bleeding in COVID-19 Patients: A Systematic Review and Meta-Analysis
Reprinted from: *Medicina* 2023, 59, 1500, doi:10.3390/medicina59081500 90

Evangelos Tsipotis, Ankith Maremanda, Laura Bowles Zeiser, Caoilfhionn Connolly, Sowmya Sharma, Sharon Dudley-Brown, et al.
Antibody Kinetics after Three Doses of SARS-CoV-2 mRNA Vaccination in Patients with Inflammatory Bowel Disease
Reprinted from: *Medicina* 2023, 59, 1487, doi:10.3390/medicina59081487 114

Vlasta Oršić Frič, Vladimir Borzan, Andrej Borzan, Izabela Kiš, Branko Dmitrović and Ivana Roksandić-Križan
Colitis as the Main Presentation of COVID-19: A Case Report
Reprinted from: *Medicina* **2023**, *59*, 576, doi:10.3390/medicina59030576 . . . . **122**

About the Editors

Daniel Paramythiotis

Daniel Paramythiotis graduated from the Medical School of Aristotle University of Thessaloniki in 1994 and received his PhD degree in 2002 (grade Excellent). He was recognized as a specialist general surgeon in 2002, and he holds a postgraduate diploma specializing in liver–biliary–pancreatic surgery from the School of Medicine of the Democritus University of Thrace. Additionally, he is an instructor of a post-graduate trauma-management program (A.T.L.S.) in Northern Greece. He trained at the University Surgery Clinics of Heidelberg and Munich as well as at St Mark's Hospital in London, participating in major surgeries of the pancreas, liver, esophagus, and colon. Daniel Paramythiotis is Full Professor of Surgery in the First Propaedeutic Department of Surgery, AHEPA University General Hospital, Aristotle University of Thessaloniki, Greece. Also, he is a member of the disciplinary board of the Medical Society of Thessaloniki, and he served as member on the board of directors for the AHEPA University General Hospital of Thessaloniki, a member of the Scientific Council of the AHEPA University General Hospital of Thessaloniki, a member of the General Assembly of School of Medicine of Aristotle University of Thessaloniki, and a member of the Committee of the Office of Education of the School of Medicine Aristotle University of Thessaloniki. His long-term service in a University Clinic and his unique abilities led him to the production of remarkable writing and research work, with numerous publications in Greek and international medical journals. Notably, he has presented as a speaker at a number of conferences and post-educational courses. Furthermore, his contributions have been recognized with numerous awards.

Eleni Karlafti

Eleni Karlafti graduated from the Medical School of Aristotle University of Thessaloniki in 2007 and earned her PhD degree in Hypertension and Obesity in 2016 (grade Excellent). In 2021, she received an MSc in «New methods and technologies in treatment of Diabetes Mellitus». Eleni was recognized as the Internal Medicine Specialist in 2017 and awarded the title of Hypertension Specialist from the European Society of Hypertension in 2020. She was recognized as the Diabetes Specialist in 2022 and received the Emergency Medicine Specialization in 2023. She is currently working in the emergency department of AHEPA University General Hospital of Thessaloniki, Aristotle University of Thessaloniki, Greece. Eleni is teaching undergraduate and postgraduate students of the Medical School of Aristotle University of Thessaloniki. She has participated in more than 25 scientific projects—as coordinator of 5—and she has published her scientific work in books and journals (over 90). Eleni has participated as an invited lecturer or coordinator in a pleiad of conferences (international and national) and received 12 awards (three international) in recognition of her scientific work and its impact.

Preface

In the last few years, the scientific world has been forced to find ways to manage the SARS-CoV-2 pandemic and its many effects. Even though COVID-19 was first considered a respiratory disease, it was found to have an extended clinical spectrum, affecting other organs. It is now identified as a systematic disease.

It is common for SARS-CoV-2 to also infect the digestive system. This type of infection in patients with COVID-19 has a wide symptom range, from asymptomatic expression to some gastrointestinal symptoms that occur with or before respiratory symptoms. Although respiratory infections are known to cause intestinal immune impairment and gastrointestinal symptoms, our knowledge around SARS-CoV-2 and its effect on the digestive system is limited.

The aim of this reprint is to evaluate and discuss the optimal management of emergency surgeries in patients with SARS-CoV-2 infection and co-infections and to explore surgeries with similarly aims from the non-COVID-19 era.

Additionally, this reprint determines the presence of SARS-CoV-2 in patients who do not have the typical respiratory symptoms, but only present with symptoms of the digestive system and to investigate the role of immature granulocytes in the early diagnosis of these patients.

Furthermore, this reprint refers to rare conditions of the digestive system and emphasizes the importance of considering these entities in the differential diagnosis of acute abdomen and discusses the preferred approach. Likewise, it includes an illustration of the spectrum of the gastrointestinal imaging findings in patients with COVID-19. Awareness of diagnostic imaging hallmarks is crucial to optimize the management of these patients.

In this reprint, we discuss the risk of new-onset liver injuries due to COVID-19 in preexisting hepatic conditions, their prognosis, severity and outcome, as well as the immunosuppressant treatments administered for COVID-19 and the possibility of reactivation of the hepatic virus.

Moreover, we refer to the drugs used during therapy of hospitalized COVID-19 patients, which have adverse side-effects of drug-induced liver injury—DILI—their diagnostic algorithm, the biomarkers that can assist in their identification, and also, the use of other drugs used for DILI therapy in an effort to control and prevent a severe long-term outcome.

Finally, this reprint punctuates the importance of vaccination against SARS-CoV-2 in chronic digestive diseases.

Daniel Paramythiotis and Eleni Karlafti
Editors

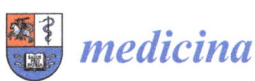

Article

Clostridium difficile Infections in an Emergency Surgical Unit from North-East Romania

Bogdan Mihnea Ciuntu [1], Gheorghe G. Balan [2], Mihaela Buna-Arvinte [1], Irina Mihaela Abdulan [3,*], Adelina Papancea [1], Ștefan Lucian Toma [4], Bogdan Veliceasa [5], Oana Viola Bădulescu [6], Gabriela Ghiga [7], Ana Maria Fătu [8], Mihai Bogdan Vascu [9], Antonia Moldovanu [9], Dan Vintilă [1] and Alin Mihai Vasilescu [1]

1. Department of General Surgery, "Grigore T. Popa" University of Medicine and Pharmacy, Universitatii Street, No. 16, 700115 Iasi, Romania; bogdan-mihnea.ciuntu@umfiasi.ro (B.M.C.); buna.mihaela@umfiasi.ro (M.B.-A.); papancea.adelina@umfiasi.ro (A.P.); dan.vintila@yahoo.com (D.V.)
2. Department of Gastroenterology, "Grigore T. Popa" University of Medicine and Pharmacy, Universitatii Street, No. 16, 700115 Iasi, Romania; gheorghe-g-balan@umfiasi.ro
3. Department of Medical Specialties I, "Grigore T. Popa" University of Medicine and Pharmacy, 700115 Iasi, Romania
4. Department of Materials Engineering and Industrial Security, Faculty of Materials Science and Engineering, Gheorghe Asachi Technical University of Iasi, 700050 Iasi, Romania; stl_toma@yahoo.com
5. Department of Traumatology and Orthopaedics, Faculty of Medicine, "Grigore T. Popa" University of Medicine and Pharmacy, 700115 Iasi, Romania; bogdan.veliceasa@umfiasi.ro
6. Department of Haematolohy, Faculty of Medicine, "Grigore T. Popa" University of Medicine and Pharmacy, 700115 Iasi, Romania; viola.badulescu@umfiasi.ro
7. Department of Mother and Child Medicine, Faculty of Medicine, "Grigore T. Popa" University of Medicine and Pharmacy, 700115 Iasi, Romania; gabriela.ghica@umfiasi.ro
8. Department of Implantology Removable Denture Technology, Discipline of Ergonomy, Faculty of Medicine, "Grigore T. Popa" University of Medicine and Pharmacy, 700115 Iasi, Romania; ana.fatu@umfiasi.ro
9. Department of Odontology, Periodontology and Fixed Prosthesis, Faculty of Medicine, "Grigore T. Popa" University of Medicine and Pharmacy, 700115 Iasi, Romania; mihai.vascu@umfiasi.ro (M.B.V.); antonia.moldovanu@umfiasi.ro (A.M.)
* Correspondence: irina.abdulan@yahoo.com

Abstract: *Background and Objectives*: Colitis with *Clostridium difficile* is an important health problem that occurs with an intensity that varies between mild and severe. Surgical interventions are required only in fulminant forms. There is little evidence regarding the best surgical intervention in these cases. *Materials and Methods*: Patients with *C. difficile* infection were identified from the two surgery clinics from the 'Saint Spiridon' Emergency Hospital Iași, Romania. Data regarding the presentation, indication for surgery, antibiotic therapy, type of toxins, and post-operative outcomes were collected over a 3-year period. *Results*: From a total of 12,432 patients admitted for emergency or elective surgery, 140 (1.12%) were diagnosed with *C. difficile* infection. The mortality rate was 14% (20 cases). Non-survivors had higher rates of lower-limb amputations, bowel resections, hepatectomy, and splenectomy. Additional surgery was necessary in 2.8% of cases because of the complications of *C. difficile* colitis. In three cases, terminal colostomy was performed and as well as one case with subtotal colectomy with ileostomy. All patients who required the second surgery died within the 30-day mortality period. *Conclusions*: In our prospective study, the incidence was increased both in cases of patients with interventions on the colon and in those requiring limb amputations. Surgical interventions are rarely required in patients with *C. difficile* colitis.

Keywords: *Clostridium difficile* infection; colitis; surgical intervention; mortality

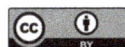

1. Introduction

Clostridium difficile is an anaerobic, sporulated Gram-positive bacillus that was discovered in 1935. Considered a rare infection until 1970, after the introduction of antibiotic treatment, the *C. difficile* infection rate increased [1]. Studies have shown that approximately

5% of adults and 15–70% of children are colonized with C. *difficile*. However, only a small portion develops the infection, being protected by normal intestinal peristalsis and an intact microbial intestinal flora [2]. Consequently, two entities of the pathology are defined: colonization (detection of bacteria without symptoms predominantly nosocomial infection) and infection (detection of toxins and symptoms) [3].

It is highly transmissible through the fecal–oral route and its exotoxins cause a spectrum of disease ranging from mild diarrhea to severe complications such as dehydration, infectious colitis, toxic megacolon, colonic perforation, sepsis, circulatory shock, and death [4]. The mortality rate increases with the severity of the infection, reaching around 34% in cases of patients admitted to the ICU [5].

As it was mentioned before, although C. *difficile* toxins were highlighted earlier by researchers, it was only in 1970 that their role in the development of pseudomembranous colitis was confirmed. This bacterium produces at least two toxins called A (TcdA) and B (TcdB). Toxin A, an enterotoxin, causes an increase in fluid secretion and inflammation in the intestinal mucosa. Toxin B, which in vitro exhibits a cytotoxic action approximately 1000 times stronger than toxin A, acts synergistically with it. While toxin A is produced by almost all strains of C. *difficile* involved in the disease, it has recently been shown that some strains secrete only toxin B [1].

In 2002, a variant of this bacterium was discovered, ribotype 027, initially in North America, later in other parts of the world. The epidemiological importance comes from the fact that it is more aggressive and contagious by synthesizing an additional toxin [6]. Until 2011, the incidence of C. *difficile* infection also increased in Romania, which correlated with the highest share determined by ribotype 027 recorded in the European Union states, approximately 70% of all cases [7].

In a country report from 2018 that analyzed the evolution of C. *difficile* infection in Romania, out of a total of 10,241 confirmed cases, 7743% (76%) were classified as healthcare-associated infections, 1931 (19%) as community infections and 567 (6%) were infections of undetermined origin [8].

Patients at highest risk for C. *difficile* infection include hospitalized individuals aged over 65 years old with recent antibiotic exposure. Pertinent explanations include depletion of protective gut flora by antibiotics and a diminished immune response to C. *difficile* due to age and medical comorbidities [9]. Most epidemics occur in the hospital setting and in long-term care facilities, but outpatient acquisition is also described [10]. The risk factors of community-acquired infections, apart from those mentioned before, are white race, cardiac disease, chronic kidney disease, and inflammatory bowel disease [11].

Active monitoring and limiting the unnecessary administration of antibiotics are key to minimizing this type of infection. The incidence rates obtained from a standard surveillance system can be used as an important indicator of the quality of healthcare. In Europe, epidemiological data on C. *difficile* infection in acute care units are derived from a few limited studies, with significant differences in study design [12].

However, antibiotic treatment cannot always resolve the effects of the infection. The surgical option is indicated in complicated C. *difficile* infection because of fulminant colitis, toxic megacolon, severe ileus, or colonic perforations. The outcome is reserved with a high mortality [13], but surgery performed before the onset of multi-system organ failure (MSOF) and hemodynamic instability could increase the rate of survival [14].

The aim of this study was to find out an updated rate of C. *difficile* infections in a large surgical clinic from the north-east of Romania considering the extent of empiric antibiotic treatments nowadays. The specifics of the clinic mainly include acute and trauma cases. At the same time, we wanted to observe if there were differences in the evolution of patients depending on the pathologies that required hospitalization, the operations performed, and the medical treatment administered, considering the fact that some pathologies required pre- and post-operative antibiotic treatment.

2. Materials and Methods

2.1. Study Design and Setting

This prospective study was conducted between September 2019 and September 2022, in the First and Second Surgery Clinic from the Emergency Hospital 'Saint Spiridon' from Iasi, Romania. Our research included the patients admitted for emergency surgeries.

2.2. Study Participants

From a total of 12,432 patients that were admitted to our clinic, we identified 140 patients who were diagnosed with post-operative *C. difficile* infection within the same hospital stay. Data regarding the age, sex, diagnostic of admission, type of surgery performed, antibiotic therapy used, type of toxins, evolution, and post-operative outcomes were collected.

2.3. Diagnosis and Laboratory Technique

In order to confirm the infection, samples were taken from freshly emitted feces in single-use containers without preservative. They were processed within a safety interval of 3 h in an external certified laboratory.

A standard amount of the diluted sample was mixed with conjugate solution 1 (contained specific monoclonal antibodies against *C. difficile* toxin A and toxin B conjugated with colored microparticles) as well as with conjugate solution 2 (contained specific anti-toxin A and anti-toxin B antibodies biotinylated).

A volume of this mixture was transferred into a dedicated window of the test box; the box contained immobilized streptavidin in the test strip and goat anti-immunoglobulin antibodies in the control strip. Specific antibodies bound to the antigen in the sample and form "sandwich" antigen–antibody complexes.

The complexes migrated through capillarity, reaching the area containing the test strip, binding to the streptavidin present in the solid phase and were visualized in the form of a black colored band, of any intensity, in the results window. In the absence of toxin A and/or B from the sample, no band was visualized. The test was validated only if a band colored black, of any intensity, was obtained in the control window.

After the diagnosis, the patients were isolated to prevent the spread of the infection.

2.4. Ethical Approval

In order to be admitted to the study, all the patients completed an informed consent form. The ethics approval was received in 2018 (no. 8404/03.05.2018 issued by the Ministry of National Education—University of Medicine and Pharmacy Gr. T. Popa—Iasi).

2.5. Statistical Methods

Data analysis was performed using SPSS 20.0 (Statistical Package for the Social Sciences, Chicago, IL, USA). For continuous data, the distribution was assessed by the Shapiro–Wilk test. Data were entered as the mean ± standard deviation, or a number with a percent frequency for continuous variables with a normal distribution. Continuous variables with normal distributions were compared using independent samples for the Student's *t*-test in the case of two samples. For continuous variables not satisfying the assumption of normality, the evaluation was done by applying nonparametric tests, i.e., the Mann–Whitney U test in the case of two samples. Results with a p-value < 0.05 were considered statistically significant.

3. Results

From a total of 12,432 patients admitted, 140 were diagnosed with *C. difficile* infection (1.12%). The average age of was 64.42 ± 16.31, 52.8% of them were men and 47.14 % women. A total of 20 (14.28%) patients died within the same hospital stay. The differences between survivors and non-survivors are illustrated in Table 1.

Table 1. Characteristics of the study group and differences between the group of survivors and the non-survivors.

	Total n = 140	Survivors n = 120	Non-Survivors n = 20	p-Value
Age (mean ± SD)	64.42 ± 16.31	63.66 ± 15.64	68.95 ± 19.76	0.18
Gender, n (%)				
Men	74 (52.86)	69 (57.5)	5 (25)	0.14
Women	66 (47.14)	51 (42.5)	15 (75)	
C. difficile toxin, n (%)				
A	20 (14.28)	17 (14.16)	3 (15)	0.92
B	5 (3.57)	4 (3.33)	1 (0.5)	0.71
A + B	115 (82.14)	99 (82.5)	16 (80)	0.78
Contact with C. difficile infection, n (%)	48 (34.28)	41 (34.16)	7 (35)	0.94
Perioperative antibiotic therapy, n (%)	53 (37.85)	42 (35)	11 (55)	0.08
Post-operative antibiotic therapy, n (%)	120 (85.71)	103 (85.83)	17 (85)	0.92
Treatment, n (%)				
Vancomycin	85 (60.71)	76 (63.33)	9 (45)	0.12
Vancomycin + Metronidazole	55 (39.28)	44 (36.66)	11 (55)	
MSOF, n (%)	25 (17.85)	6 (5)	19 (95)	<0.00001
Previous multiple hospitalizations, n (%)	68 (48.57)	56 (46.66)	12 (60)	0.038

MSOF-Multiple systems organ failure.

From all the patients, 34.28% (n = 48) were contacts with at least one patient that was positive for *C. difficile* infection. Both toxins were identified after surgery in 82.14% (n = 115), with no significant differences between survivors and non-survivors.

Most of the patients, 85% (n = 120) were admitted directly to our clinic and 15% (n = 20) of cases were initially admitted in other medical specialties. Complicated forms of the infection were found in 17.85% (n = 25) due to multiple systems organ failure.

Neoplasm of the colon was the main diagnostis in 17.85% (n = 25), 10 % were acute cholecystitis, incisional hernia, and gangrene of the lower limb (Figure 1).

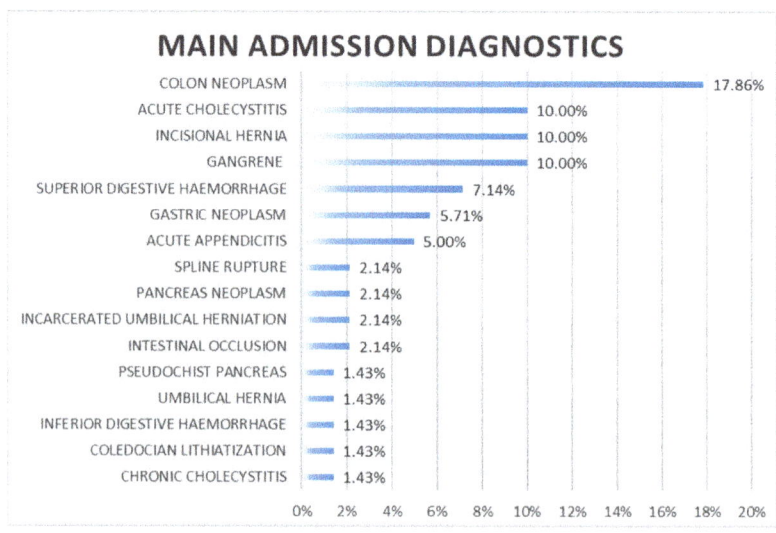

Figure 1. Main admission diagnostics.

Regarding the election of the medical treatment, approximately two thirds received monotherapy (Vancomycin) and one third double had antibiotic therapy (vancomycin and metronidazole). The dosage we used for vancomycin was 125 mg PO q6hr and for metronidazole, 500 mg PO q8hr for 10 days. We noted a difference between treatments in the case of survivors (Table 2).

Table 2. Election of the antibiotic therapy.

	Vancomycin	Vancomycin and Metronidazole	p-Value
Survivors, n (%)	76 (63.33)	44 (36.66)	0.000002
Non-survivors, n (%)	9 (45)	11 (55)	0.53

Analyzing the surgical interventions, there were significant differences between survivors and non-survivors. There were higher rates of lower-limb amputations, bowel resections, hepatectomy, and splenectomy in the survivors (Table 3).

Table 3. Types of surgical interventions.

Type of Surgery	Total n = 140	Survivors n = 120	Non-Survivors n = 20	p-Value
Gastric or esophageal operations, n (%)	21 (15)	21 (17.5)	0 (0)	-
Bowel resection or repair, n (%)	47 (33.57)	40 (30)	7 (35)	0.78
Hepatectomy, n (%)	2 (1.4)	1 (0.83)	1 (5)	0.56
Splenectomy, n (%)	3 (2.14)	2 (1.66)	1 (5)	0.14
Pancreatectomy, n (%)	5 (3.57)	5 (4.16)	0 (0)	-
Cholecystectomy, n (%)	19 (13.57)	18 (15)	1 (5)	0.22
Lower-extremity amputation, n (%)	16 (11.42)	10 (8.3)	6 (30)	**0.04**
Hernia, n (%)	19 (13.57)	19 (15.8)	0 (0)	-
Other, n (%)	4 (2.85)	4 (3.33)	0 (0)	-

Surgery was necessary in four patients (2.8%) because of the complications of *C. difficile* colitis, due to toxic megacolon and (n = 3) and bowel perforation (n = 1).

In four of the cases, emergency surgical intervention was needed due to infection complications. Of these, in three cases, terminal colostomy was performed and in one case subtotal colectomy with ileostomy. All patients were admitted to the intensive care unit post-operatively with a mean stay of 10 days.

The total mortality rate in *C. difficile* infections was 14% (n = 20), but all patients who required additional surgery died within the 30-day mortality period.

4. Discussion

The present research is a prospective one in which we collected information over a 3-year period. From 12,432 patients admitted, 1.12% were diagnosed with *C. difficile* infection. Previous studies have reported an incidence of up to 7.8%, reaching three times higher values in cases of patients with colon surgery [15,16].

More than half of the deceased patients (60%) had a history of multiple hospitalizations, with statistically significant differences when compared to the surviving patients. The data obtained are consistent with the data from the literature, considering that healthcare exposures before the hospitalization may increase the risk for *C. difficile* infection [17].

Two large clostridial glucosylating toxins, toxin A (TcdA) and toxin B (TcdB), are involved in the pathogenesis of *C. difficile*. There are some strains that produce a third toxin, the binary toxin *C. difficile* transferase, which can also contribute to *C. difficile* virulence and disease. These toxins act on the colonic epithelium and immune cells and induce a complex cascade of cellular events that result in fluid secretion, inflammation, and tissue damage, which are the hallmark features of the disease. In our study, 82.14% presented both toxins, these being the majority both in the case of the survivors and non-survivors.

In a large-scale study that followed patients from 52 hospitals from Michigan, USA, between 2012 and 2013, Abdelsattar et al. showed that the highest rate of *C. difficile* infection occurred after the interventions of amputation of the lower limbs, bowel resection, and esophageal and gastric interventions [18]. In our study, the results were slightly reversed with the highest percentage being interventions on the colon followed by amputations and eso-gastric interventions.

Moreover, we observed statistically significant differences only in the case of limb amputation operations (30% versus 8.3%). It is worth mentioning that in cases of patients with a bad outcome, there was a higher rate of bowel resection, 35% compared to 30% in the case of survivors.

In the treatment approach to *C. difficile* infection, clinicians aim to cure both the first episode and to reduce the risk of recurrences. In the recently updated Infectious Diseases Society of America/Society for Healthcare Epidemiology of America (IDSA/SHEA) guidelines and the updated European Society of Clinical Microbiology and Infectious Diseases (ESCMID) guidance document, fidaxomicin is now recommended as the first treatment option over vancomycin for both the first episode and for relapse *C. difficile* infection. Although vancomycin is still a suitable alternative to fidaxomicin, specific focus was placed on the improved results and reduced risk of relapse observed with fidaxomicin compared to vancomycin [19,20]. Consequently, the new recommendations converge on a main idea: to consider fidaxomicin first, considering the global benefits of the patient, if feasible. Regarding the last aspect, fidaxomicin is more expensive than vancomycin, so accessibility remains reduced in multiple hospitals. ESCMID guide through a good practice statement mentions that when fidaxomicin is unavailable or unfeasible, vancomycin remains a suitable alternative.

Referring to the treatment options used in the surgery clinics from our study, the high cost of this macrolide makes it difficult to be used as the first option in the treatment of this type of infection for the time being. Consequently, the treatment options used in that period were metronidazole and vancomycin.

The choice of treatment—monotherapy or bitherapy—did not present differences between the two categories, survivors and non-survivors, that followed the treatments according to current recommendations [21]. However, in the case of survivors, monotherapy was preferred in 63.33% of cases ($p = 0.000002$), while in the case of those with a bad outcome, double association was chosen in 55% of cases.

Several studies have shown that a prophylactic dose given before surgery is associated with substantially reduced rates of wound infection and post-operative sepsis, especially in the case of bowel interventions [22,23]. Additionally, in these cases, the risk of developing *C. difficile* infection was outweighed by the benefit of avoiding a wound infection. It should be noted that there were also other pathologies/surgical interventions that required antibiotic treatment (gangrene of the lower limb) in the case of the patients included in our study.

Of the 140 patients, 37.85% had antibiotic treatment pre-operatively, and 85.71% after the surgical intervention, with a slightly higher rate in the case of patients with a bad outcome. There were no significant differences between the two groups. Currently, there is no consensus on the pre-operative administration of antibiotics, but a short course for bowel preparation is insisted upon, if necessary, since prolonged treatment can be a risk factor for developing *C. difficile* infection in patients undergoing colorectal surgery [24].

Post-operatively, the unfavorable evolution of the symptoms appeared in 17.85% of the cases. Multiple systems organ failure occurred in 5% of the survivors, the percentage reaching up to 95% in the case of patients who died. Factors such as advanced age, the presence of comorbidities, and prolonged previous treatment with PPIs can hinder the evolution of the infection, despite the initiation of prompt antibiotic treatment [25]. Several reported cases showed that even after using all the available resources, evolution can be lethal. In addition, when multiple system organ failure is present, survival is not positively influenced by radical intervention or subtotal colectomy [26,27].

C. difficile has become a significant public health threat in the past decade, largely due to the emergence/selection of hypervirulent strains that persist in healthcare-associated settings and cause more severe infections [28]. These strains are now being associated with disease in healthy individuals who are not part of the population considered to be at risk [29,30].

The presence of the infection and the growing aggressiveness of the pathogen influence the post-operative evolution of the patients. Moreover, some cases cannot be solved by antibiotic treatment and worsen, requiring emergency interventions, with extensive bowel resections, whose evolution is most often unfavorable. These cases especially appear in tertiary, large, university hospitals, where the number of performed surgeries has increased, but also the diversity and complexity of the cases are greater.

C. difficile infection occurs as a chronic or an acute illness with intensity varying from mild to severe. Most cases can be managed with antibiotics and supportive care. Surgical intervention in terms of colectomy is rarely required in patients with *C. difficile* colitis. However, when the patient presents with fulminant disease, the early decision to perform surgery is imperative for survival. Performed before the total morpho-functional degradation of the colon and the development of complications, surgery has lower rates of complications and post-operative lethality.

The current standard of care is subtotal colectomy. However, loop ileostomy with vancomycin enemas delivered into the colonic mucosa has been described as a viable option on selected patients [12].

In our study, 2.8% of the cases needed additional surgery because of the complications of *C. difficile* infection. The intervention rate is slightly higher compared to other studies, but the comparison is difficult considering the small groups studied in previous research [31].

It is important to emphasize that multidisciplinary collaboration and early surgical intervention can improve the outcome of patients with fulminant infection.

Fulminant *C. difficile* colitis remains associated with exceptionally high mortality following surgical intervention. The adoption of loop ileostomy as a valid alternative to conventional surgical interventions, such as total colectomy, has more than doubled over the past few years. The data in this study corroborated prior findings regarding equivalent outcomes between both procedures. While the results from randomized clinical trials and a better understanding of functional outcomes are both needed, it appears that loop ileostomy is a viable alternative for acute care surgeons during management of fulminant colitis [32,33].

The strength of the study is that it is a prospective one. The limitations consist of the small batch of patients from a single center, the incomplete medical history, unclear previous treatment with empiric antibiotherapy, and self-prescribed PPI intake.

5. Conclusions

C. difficile infection remains a major public health problem, especially in surgical wards. In our research, the incidence was increased both in the case of patients with interventions on the colon, and in those requiring limb amputations. The low number of patients who developed the infection is a positive aspect, but we are currently considering follow-up over a longer period of time to be able to include a larger number of patients, also from other regional surgical centers. Thus, we will be able to have an objective and more extensive perspective on the subject.

Clear and rigorous assessment of the risk factors for *C. difficile* infection is recommended to adjust pre-operative care and surgical management. Further studies are needed to complete our findings and a multidisciplinary approach is mandatory when it comes to proper prevention and treatment.

Author Contributions: Conceptualization, M.B.-A.; methodology, B.M.C.; software, G.G.B. and A.P.; validation, B.M.C. and M.B.-A.; formal analysis, O.V.B., B.V.; investigation, G.G. and A.M.F.; resources, B.M.C.; data curation, M.B.V. and A.M.; writing—original draft preparation, I.M.A.; writing—review and editing, B.M.C.; visualization, A.P. and Ș.L.T.; supervision, A.M.V. and D.V.; project administration. All authors had an equal contribution to this manuscript. All authors have read and agreed to the published version of the manuscript.

Funding: This research received no external funding.

Institutional Review Board Statement: The study was conducted in accordance with the Declaration of Helsinki and approved by the Institutional Review Board (or Ethics Committee) of University of Medicine and Pharmacy Gr. T. Popa—Iasi (protocol code 8404) for studies involving humans approved on 3 May 2018.

Informed Consent Statement: Informed consent was obtained from all subjects involved in the study.

Data Availability Statement: The data published in this research are available on request from the first author and corresponding authors.

Conflicts of Interest: The authors declare no conflict of interest.

References

1. Smits, W.K.; Lyras, D.; Lacy, D.B.; Wilcox, M.H.; Kuijper, E.J. *Clostridium difficile* infection. *Nat. Rev. Dis. Prim.* **2016**, *2*, 16020. [CrossRef]
2. Baktash, A.; Terveer, E.M.; Zwittink, R.D.; Hornung, B.V.H.; Corver, J.; Kuijper, E.J.; Smits, W.K. Mechanistic insights in the success of fecal microbiota transplants for the treatment of *Clostridium difficile* infections. *Front. Microbiol.* **2018**, *9*, 1242. [CrossRef] [PubMed]
3. Knight, D.R.; Elliott, B.; Chang, B.J.; Perkins, T.T.; Riley, T.V. Diversity and Evolution in the Genome of *Clostridium difficile*. *Clin. Microbiol. Rev.* **2015**, *28*, 721–741. [CrossRef] [PubMed]
4. D'Aoust, J.; Battat, R.; Bessissow, T. Management of inflammatory bowel disease with *Clostridium difficile* infection. *World J. Gastroenterol.* **2017**, *23*, 4986–5003. [CrossRef]
5. Marttila-Vaara, M.; Ylipalosaari, P.; Kauma, H. *Clostridium difficile* infections in teaching hospital in northern Finland. *BMC Infect. Dis.* **2019**, *19*, 48. [CrossRef] [PubMed]
6. Vincent, J.L.; Rello, J.; Marshall, J.; Silva, E.; Anzueto, A.; Martin, C.D.; Moreno, R.; Lipman, J.; Gomersall, C.; Sakr, Y.; et al. International study of the prevalence and outcomes of infection in intensive care units. *J. Am. Med. Assoc.* **2009**, *302*, 2323–2329. [CrossRef]
7. Rafila, A.; Indra, A.; Popescu, G.A.; Wewalka, G.; Allerberger, F.; Benea, S.; Badicut, I.; Aschbacher, R.; Huhulescu, S. Occurrence of *Clostridium difficile* infections due to PCR ribotype 027 in Bucharest, Romania. *J. Infect. Dev. Ctries.* **2014**, *8*, 694–698. [CrossRef]
8. Krutova, M.; Kinross, P.; Barbut, F.; Hajdu, A.; Wilcox, M.; Kuijper, E.; Allerberger, F.; Delmée, M.; Van Broeck, J.; Vatcheva-Dobrevska, R.; et al. How to: Surveillance of *Clostridium difficile* infections. *Clin. Microbiol. Infect.* **2018**, *24*, 46. [CrossRef]
9. Analiza Evoluției Infecției cu Clostridium Difficile în Spitalele din România. 2018. Available online: https://www.cnscbt.ro (accessed on 23 January 2023).
10. Jachowicz, E.; Pac, A.; Różańska, A.; Gryglewska, B.; Wojkowska-Mach, J. Post-Discharge *Clostridioides difficile* Infection after Arthroplasties in Poland, Infection Prevention and Control as the Key Element of Prevention of C. difficile Infections. *Int. J. Environ. Res. Public Health* **2022**, *19*, 3155. [CrossRef]
11. Crobach, M.J.; Planche, T.; Eckert, C.; Barbut, F.; Terveer, E.M.; Dekkers, O.M.; Wilcox, M.H.; Kuijper, E.J. European Society of Clinical Microbiology and Infectious Diseases: Update of the diagnostic guidance document for *Clostridium difficile* infection. *Clin. Microbiol. Infect.* **2016**, *22* (Suppl. S4), S63–S81. [CrossRef]
12. Guh, A.Y.; Adkins, S.H.; Li, Q.; Bulens, S.N.; Farley, M.M.; Smith, Z.; Holzbauer, S.M.; Whitten, T.; Phipps, E.C.; Hancock, E.B.; et al. Risk factors for community-associated *Clostridium difficile* infection in adults: A case-control study. *Open Forum Infect. Dis.* **2017**, *4*, ofx171. [CrossRef] [PubMed]
13. Crobach, M.J.T.; Vernon, J.J.; Loo, V.G.; Kong, L.Y.; Péchiné, S.; Wilcox, M.H.; Kuijper, E.J. Understanding *Clostridium difficile* Colonization. *Clin. Microbiol. Rev.* **2018**, *31*, e00021-17. [CrossRef]
14. Desai, J.; Elnaggar, M.; Hanfy, A.A.; Doshi, R. Toxic Megacolon: Background, Pathophysiology, Management Challenges and Solutions. *Clin. Exp. Gastroenterol.* **2020**, *13*, 203–210. [CrossRef]
15. Gateau, C.; Couturier, J.; Coia, J.; Barbut, F. How to: Diagnose infection caused by *Clostridium difficile*. *Clin. Microbiol. Infect.* **2018**, *24*, 463–468. [CrossRef] [PubMed]
16. Yeom, C.H.; Cho, M.M.; Baek, S.K.; Bae, O.S. Risk factors for the development of *Clostridium difficile*-associated colitis after colorectal cancer surgery. *J. Korean Soc. Coloproctol.* **2010**, *26*, 329–333. [CrossRef] [PubMed]
17. Kelly, C.P.; LaMont, J.T. *Clostridium difficile*—More difficult than ever. *N. Engl. J. Med.* **2008**, *359*, 1932–1940. [CrossRef] [PubMed]
18. Miller, A.C.; Sewell, D.K.; Segre, A.M.; Pemmaraju, S.V.; Polgreen, P.M. Risk for *Clostridioides difficile* Infection among Hospitalized Patients Associated with Multiple Healthcare Exposures Prior to Admission. *J. Infect. Dis.* **2021**, *224*, 684–694. [CrossRef]
19. Abdelsattar, Z.M.; Krapohl, G.; Alrahmani, L.; Banerjee, M.; Krell, R.W.; Wong, S.L.; Campbell, D.A.; Aronoff, D.M.; Hendren, S. Postoperative Burden of Hospital-Acquired *Clostridium difficile* Infection. *Infect. Control. Hosp. Epidemiol.* **2015**, *36*, 40–46. [CrossRef]
20. Johnson, S.; Lavergne, V.; Skinner, A.M.; Gonzales-Luna, A.J.; Garey, K.W.; Kelly, C.P.; Wilcox, M.H. Clinical Practice Guideline by the Infectious Diseases Society of America (IDSA) and Society for Healthcare Epidemiology of America (SHEA): 2021 Focused Update Guidelines on Management of *Clostridioides difficile* Infection in Adults. *Clin. Infect. Dis.* **2021**, *73*, 755–757. [CrossRef]

21. van Prehn, J.; Reigadas, E.; Vogelzang, E.H.; Bouza, E.; Hristea, A.; Guery, B.; Krutova, M.; Noren, T.; Allerberger, F.; Coia, J.E.; et al. European Society of Clinical Microbiology and Infectious Diseases: 2021 update on the treatment guidance document for *Clostridioides difficile* infection in adults. *Clin. Microbiol. Infect.* **2021**, *27* (Suppl. S2), S1–S21. [CrossRef]
22. Debast, S.B.; Bauer, M.P.; Kuijper, E.J. ESCMID European Society of Clinical Microbiology and Infectious Diseases: Update of the treatment guidance document for *Clostridium difficile* infection. *Clin. Microbiol. Infect.* **2014**, *20* (Suppl. S2), 1–26. [CrossRef] [PubMed]
23. Lewis, R.T. Oral versus systemic antibiotic prophylaxis in elective colon surgery: A randomized study and meta-analysis send a message from the 1990s. *Can. J. Surg.* **2002**, *45*, 173–180. [PubMed]
24. Clarke, J.S.; Condon, R.E.; Bartlett, J.G.; Gorbach, S.L.; Nichols, R.L.; Ochi, S. Preoperative oral antibiotics reduce septic complications of colon operations: Results of prospective, randomized, double-blind clinical study. *Ann. Surg.* **1977**, *186*, 251–259. [CrossRef] [PubMed]
25. Krapohl, G.L.; Phillips, L.; Campbell, D.A.; Hendren, S., Jr.; Banerjee, M.; Metzger, B.; Morris, A.M. Bowel preparation for colectomy and risk of *Clostridium difficile* infection. *Dis. Colon Rectum* **2011**, *54*, 810–817. [CrossRef]
26. Lessa, F.C.; Mu, Y.; Bamberg, W.M.; Beldavs, Z.G.; Dumyati, G.K.; Dunn, J.R.; Farley, M.M.; Holzbauer, S.M.; Meek, J.I.; Phipps, E.C.; et al. Burden of Clostridium difficile infection in the United States. *N. Engl. J. Med.* **2015**, *372*, 825–834. [CrossRef]
27. Halabi, W.J.; Nguyen, V.Q.; Carmichael, J.C.; Pigazzi, A.; Stamos, M.J.; Mills, S. *Clostridium difficile* colitis in the United States: A decade of trends, outcomes, risk factors for colectomy, and mortality after colectomy. *J. Am. Coll. Surg.* **2013**, *217*, 802–812. [CrossRef]
28. Bermejo, C.; Maseda, E.; Salgado, P.; Gabilondo, G.; Gilsanz, F. Shock séptico debido a la infección por *Clostridium difficile* adquirida en la comunidad. Estudio de un caso y revisión de la literatura. *Rev. Española Anestesiol. Reanim.* **2014**, *61*, 219–222. [CrossRef]
29. Shen, A. *Clostridium difficile* Toxins: Mediators of Inflammation. *J. Innate Immun.* **2012**, *4*, 149–158. [CrossRef]
30. Birgand, G.; Blanckaert, K.; Carbonne, A.; Coignard, B.; Barbut, F.; Eckert, C.; Grandbastien, B.; Kadi, Z.; Astagneau, P. Investigation of a large outbreak of *Clostridium difficile* PCR-ribotype 027 infections in northern France, 2006–2007 and associated clusters in 2008–2009. *Eurosurveillance* **2010**, *15*, 19597. [CrossRef]
31. Stelzmueller, I.; Goegele, H.; Biebl, M.; Wiesmayr, S.; Berger, N.; Tabarelli, W.; Ruttmann, E.; Albright, J.; Margreiter, R.; Fille, M.; et al. *Clostridium difficile* colitis in solid organ transplantationea single-center experience. *Dig. Dis. Sci.* **2007**, *52*, 3231–3236. [CrossRef]
32. McMaster-Baxter, N.L.; Musher, D.M. *Clostridium difficile*: Recent epidemiologic findings and advances in therapy. *Pharmacotherapy* **2007**, *27*, 1029–1039. [CrossRef] [PubMed]
33. Juo, Y.Y.; Sanaiha, Y.; Jabaji, Z.; Benharash, P. Trends in Diverting Loop Ileostomy vs Total Abdominal Colectomy as Surgical Management for *Clostridium Difficile* Colitis. *JAMA Surg.* **2019**, *154*, 899–906. [CrossRef] [PubMed]

Disclaimer/Publisher's Note: The statements, opinions and data contained in all publications are solely those of the individual author(s) and contributor(s) and not of MDPI and/or the editor(s). MDPI and/or the editor(s) disclaim responsibility for any injury to people or property resulting from any ideas, methods, instructions or products referred to in the content.

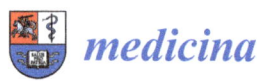

Article

Could an Increased Percentage of Immature Granulocytes Accompanying Dyspepsia Predict COVID-19?

Kadir Gisi [1,*], Sukru Gungor [2], Murat Ispiroglu [1] and Bulent Kantarceken [1]

[1] Department of Gastroenterology, Sutcu Imam University, Kahramanmaras 46050, Turkey
[2] Department of Pediatric Gastroenterology, Sutcu Imam University, Kahramanmaras 46050, Turkey
* Correspondence: kadirgisi@gmail.com

Abstract: *Background and Aim*: Although vaccination practices continue at a fast pace around the world, the severe acute respiratory syndrome coronavirus 2 (SARS-CoV-2) still threatens people's lives. In this study, we aimed to determine the presence of SARS-CoV-2 in patients who do not have the typical symptoms of the novel coronavirus disease 2019 (COVID-19), but only present with dyspepsia, and to investigate the role of immature granulocytes in the early diagnosis of these patients. *Material and Methods*: Adult and pediatric patients suffering from dyspepsia were included in the study. The patients were divided into two groups, "positive" and "negative", based on their SARS-CoV-2 polymerase chain reaction test results. Immature granulocyte count (IG), immature granulocyte percentage (IG%), C-reactive protein (CRP), and neutrophil-to-lymphocyte ratio (NLR) values were recorded. *Results*: A total of 238 patients, including 25 (10.5%) pediatric and 213 (89.5%) adult patients, were included in the study. A total of 2 (8%) pediatric patients and 17 (7.9%) adult patients tested positive for SARS-CoV-2. The IG, IG%, and CRP parameters were significantly higher in the SARS-CoV-2-positive patients compared to the SARS-CoV-2-negative patients. The optimal cut-off value predictive of COVID-19 infection was determined to be ≥ 0.650 (sensitivity: 52.6% and specificity: 95.5%, $p = 0.001$) for IG%. *Conclusions*: It should be noted that dyspepsia may also be a COVID-19 symptom. IG% values, which can be determined with a hemogram test, a cheap and easily accessible test, may be a warning in the early detection of patients who do not have the typical symptoms of COVID-19.

Keywords: COVID-19; digestive symptom; dyspepsia; immature granulocyte

Citation: Gisi, K.; Gungor, S.; Ispiroglu, M.; Kantarceken, B. Could an Increased Percentage of Immature Granulocytes Accompanying Dyspepsia Predict COVID-19? *Medicina* 2022, 58, 1460. https://doi.org/10.3390/medicina58101460

Academic Editors: Daniel Paramythiotis and Eleni Karlafti

Received: 1 September 2022
Accepted: 12 October 2022
Published: 15 October 2022

Publisher's Note: MDPI stays neutral with regard to jurisdictional claims in published maps and institutional affiliations.

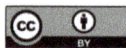

Copyright: © 2022 by the authors. Licensee MDPI, Basel, Switzerland. This article is an open access article distributed under the terms and conditions of the Creative Commons Attribution (CC BY) license (https://creativecommons.org/licenses/by/4.0/).

1. Introduction

Coronavirus pneumonia cases caused by the severe acute respiratory syndrome coronavirus 2 (SARS-CoV-2) broke out in the city of Wuhan in the Hubei province of China in early December 2019 and then spread rapidly all around the world [1]. The first novel coronavirus disease 2019 (COVID-19) case in Turkey was documented on 11 March 2020, and the pandemic was declared on the same day by the World Health Organization [2]. As occurred all around the world, immediately after the first case was declared in Turkey, changes and restrictions began to be implemented in daily life as the spread of the virus increased. COVID-19 acts similar to a systemic disease with a variable range of severity, from the asymptomatic clinical form to respiratory failure and increased mortality. COVID-19 is characterized by interstitial pneumonia and vascular damage that may lead to severe adverse outcomes, and sometimes it can be fatal [3,4]. Studies have shown that 1/10 of COVID-19 patients may only have gastrointestinal symptoms without any respiratory symptoms, which will delay their diagnosis [5]. Among the gastrointestinal symptoms identified in adult COVID-19 patients, diarrhea is the most common, followed by nausea/vomiting, and abdominal pain, and vomiting is reported to be the most common symptom in pediatric patients [6].

Moreover, restrictions upon daily life have led to stress and anxiety in people. Since dyspepsia is a stress-sensitive disorder, stress and anxiety are known to trigger and exacerbate dyspepsia [7]. A complete blood count (hemogram) is one of the commonly requested tests for patients admitted to adult and pediatric gastroenterology outpatient clinics with the complaint of increased dyspepsia [8]. Immature granulocytes (IG), which can be measured in complete blood counts, are the common name used for granulocyte (neutrophil) precursors, namely myelocytes, promyelocytes, and metamyelocytes, which are not found in peripheral blood except for during the neonatal period. IG counts and immature granulocyte percentages (IG%) can easily be obtained by performing a routine complete blood count test, thanks to technological advancements in automated hemogram devices [7]. The detection of immature granulocytes in peripheral blood is an indicator of bone marrow activation and severe infection. In recent studies, immature granulocytes have been shown to be an effective marker for predicting infection severity [9,10]. Finally, given the dynamic characteristic of the COVID-19 pandemic, the relationship between the prognosis of SARS-CoV-2 infection and digestive symptoms is still a matter of debate [11]. Additionally, in those patients with digestive symptoms, there are currently no early diagnostic markers to alert the clinician in simple laboratory tests unless the clinician suspects SARS-CoV-2 infection.

In this study, we aimed to determine the presence of SARS-CoV-2 infection in patients who did not have the typical symptoms of COVID-19 but only presented with dyspepsia and investigate the role of immature granulocytes in the early diagnosis of such patients.

2. Material and Methods

Patients presenting to pediatric and adult gastroenterology outpatient clinics with the complaint of persistent dyspepsia between August 2020 and December 2020 were included in the study. The demographic and laboratory data of the included patients were retrospectively screened and recorded.

All procedures performed in the studies involving human participants were performed in accordance with the ethical standards of the institutional and/or national research committee and the 1964 Declaration of Helsinki and its later amendments or comparable ethical standards. Approval was obtained from the local ethics committee of Sutcu Imam University before starting the study, with a decision date of 25 January 2021, session 2021/04, no. 10.

2.1. Inclusion Criteria

Pediatric and adult patients who had dyspeptic complaints resistant to diet and medical treatment, who had no complaints other than dyspepsia, who were scheduled for endoscopy, and who underwent COVİD-19 PCR tests were included in the study.

2.2. Exclusion Criteria

Patients who underwent endoscopy with indications other than resistant dyspeptic complaints, such as variceal bleeding, foreign body ingestion, and corrosive substance ingestion, and patients who had not taken a PCR test for COVID-19 were excluded from the study.

2.3. Laboratory Data Evaluated in the Study

The results of SARS-CoV-2 Polymerase Chain Reaction (PCR) tests, complete blood counts, white blood cell counts (WBCs), neutrophils, lymphocytes, hemoglobin levels, immature granulocyte counts, immature granulocyte percentages, and C-reactive protein (CRP) tests, which were routinely checked before endoscopy, were recorded.

2.4. Groups

The patients were divided into two groups (SARS-CoV-2 positive vs. SARS-CoV-2 negative), based on their PCR test results. Demographic and laboratory data were compared for these two groups.

2.5. Complete Blood Count Data Analysis

The complete blood count results were studied using an automated hematological analyzer (XN 3000; Sysmex Corp., Kobe, Japan), and WBC counts, neutrophil counts, lymphocyte counts, IG counts, and IG% values were measured. Neutrophil-to-lymphocyte ratios (NLR) were calculated manually. IG% was calculated as the ratio of the IG count value to the white blood cell count value.

2.6. SARS-CoV-2 PCR Analysis

Nasal and pharyngeal swab samples collected from the patients were examined with the CFX96 Touch Real-Time Polymerase Chain Reaction (RT-PCR) detection system using the Bio-speedy (Bioeksen) RT-PCR kit provided by the Turkish Ministry of Health.

2.7. Statistical Analysis

The statistical analyses were performed using statistical software (SPSS 22 for Windows, Chicago). Descriptive statistics are expressed as mean ± standard deviation for the continuous variables and as percentages (%) for the categorical variables. The chi-squared test and the Fisher's exact test were conducted for the categorical variables. The Shapiro–Wilk test was performed to check the normality of the distribution of the data for the continuous variables. The independent samples t-test was used to determine the mean differences of a dependent variable between two independent groups and whether there was a significant difference in the normally distributed parameters. The Mann–Whitney U test was used to compare the nonnormally distributed continuous variables. Correlation analysis was conducted to show the direction and strength of the relationship between two numeric variables. If the data were distributed normally, the Pearson correlation coefficient was preferred, whereas the Spearman's Rank correlation coefficient was preferred for the nonnormally distributed data. The numeric data are given as median ± standard deviation (minimum–maximum values), and the categorical data are shown as frequencies (n) and percentages (%). In the analyses, $p < 0.05$ was considered statistically significant.

We performed an ROC curve analysis to determine the best cut-off values of the hematological parameters that could predict the development of COVID-19 infection. We conducted a risk analysis with logistic regression according to the cut-off values that we found. Results with a p-value of <0.05 were considered statistically significant.

3. Results

A total of 238 patients, including 25 (10.5%) pediatric and 213 (89.5%) adult patients, were included in the study. The mean age of the patients was 41.08 ± 19.16 years. The mean age of the pediatric patients was 9.35 ± 5.37, and the mean age of the adult patients was 44.81 ± 16.57. A total of 11 (44%) of the pediatric patients were female, and 14 (56%) were male, while 95 (44.6%) of the adult patients were female, and 118 (55.4%) were male. A total of 2 (8%) pediatric patients and 17 (7.9%) adult patients were determined to be positive for SARS-CoV-2. There was no significant difference in terms of sex or age distributions between the patients with and without SARS-CoV-2 ($p = 0.482$, $p = 0.269$, respectively). A total of 100 (45.7%) of the SARS-CoV-2-negative patients were female, and 119 (54.3%) were male. A total of 6 (31.6%) of the SARS-CoV-2-positive patients were female, and 13 (68.4%) were male. There was no significant difference in terms of sex or age between the patients with and without SARS-CoV-2 infection ($p = 0.236$, $p = 0.269$, respectively) (Table 1).

Table 1. Comparison of laboratory data of patients with and without SARS-CoV-2 infection.

	SARS-CoV-2 Negative All Patients (219)	SARS-CoV-2 Positive All Patients (19)	
	n (%)	n (%)	p *
Gender			
Female	100 (45.7)	6 (31.6)	0.236
Male	119 (54.3)	13 (68.4)	
	Mean ± SD	Mean ± SD	p **
Age	41.45 ± 19.15	36.41 ± 19.15	0.269
WBC (10^9 L)	7.80 ± 2.83	7.42 ± 2.52	0.637
Hb (g/dl)	13.28 ± 4.24	12.41 ± 3.08	0.478
Neutrophil (10^9 L)	4.65 ± 2.51	4.19 ± 2.02	0.513
Lymphocyte (10^9 L)	2.24 ± 1.10	2.13 ± 0.97	0.739
NLR	2.53 ± 2.01	2.68 ± 1.51	0.752
IG (10^9 L)	0.033 ± 0.061	0.221 ± 0.275	0.008
IG%	0.306 ± 0.177	0.935 ± 1.249	0.042
CRP (mg/L)	5.13 ± 5.04	21.11 ± 31.92	0.043

Statistics: * Crosstabs chi-squared tests, ** Independent samples *t*-test. Abbreviations: WBC: White blood cell count; Hb: Hemoglobin; NLR: Neutrophil-to-lymphocyte ratio; IG: Immature granulocyte; IG%: Immature granulocyte percentage; CRP: C-reactive protein.

There was no significant difference between the SARS-CoV-2-positive and the SARS-CoV-2-negative groups in terms of their WBC, Hb, neutrophil, lymphocyte or NLR values ($p = 0.637$, $p = 0.478$, $p = 0.513$, $p = 0.739$, and $p = 0.752$, respectively). The IG, IG%, and CRP parameter values were statistically significantly higher in the SARS-CoV-2-positive patients in comparison to the SARS-CoV-2-negative patients ($p = 0.008$, $p = 0.042$, and $p = 0.043$, respectively) (Table 1).

There was no statistically significant difference in terms of WBC or NLR values between the SARS-CoV-2-positive and -negative pediatric patients ($p = 0.847$ and $p = 0.856$, respectively). The CRP, IG, and IG% values were statistically significantly higher in the SARS-CoV-2-positive pediatric patients compared to the SARS-CoV-2-negative pediatric patients ($p < 0.001$, $p = 0.046$, and $p < 0.001$, respectively). Additionally, there was no statistically significant difference in terms of WBC or NLR values between the SARS-CoV-2-positive and -negative adult patients ($p = 0.849$ and $p = 0.850$, respectively). However, the CRP, IG, and IG% values were statistically significantly higher in the SARS-CoV-2-positive adult patients compared to the SARS-CoV-2-negative adult patients ($p = 0.008$, $p = 0.014$, and $p = 0.009$, respectively) (Table 2). The correlations between the CRP, IG, and IG% values, which were higher in the SARS-CoV-2-positive patient group, were evaluated with the Pearson correlation test. Accordingly, there was a weakly positive significant correlation between CRP and GI values (r: 0.279, $p = 0.014$), and there was a statistically significant positive correlation between CRP and IG% values (r: 0.892 $p < 0.001$) (Table 3).

Table 2. Comparison of laboratory data in pediatric and adult patients according to the presence of SARS-CoV-2.

	Pediatric SARS-CoV-2			Adult SARS-CoV-2		
	Negative	Positive	p	Negative	Positive	p
CRP (Mean ± SD)	4.77 ± 3.69	80.5 ± 91.21	<0.001	5.36 ± 5.80	14.13 ± 11.58	0.008
WBC (10^9 L) (Mean ± SD)	8.96 ± 3.21	8.47 ± 6.25	0.847	7.39 ± 2.58	7.24 ± 1.92	0.849
NLR (Mean ± SD)	2.11 ± 1.72	1.88 ± 1.71	0.856	2.67 ± 2.09	2.78 ± 1.52	0.850
IG (10^9 L) (Mean ± SD)	0.062 ± 0.113	0.23 ± 0.007	0.046	0.023 ± 0.018	0.220 ± 0.291	0.014
IG% (Mean ± SD)	0.304 ± 0.196	3.800 ± 2.687	<0.001	0.307 ± 0.172	0.598 ± 0.398	0.009

Statistics: Independent samples *t*-test. Abbreviations: WBC: White blood cell count; Hb: Hemoglobin; NLR: Neutrophil-to-lymphocyte ratio; IG: Immature granulocyte; IG%: Immature granulocyte percentage; CRP: C-reactive protein.

Table 3. Evaluation of correlation between CRP, IG, and IG% values.

		IG	IG%
CRP	r	0.279	0.892
	p	0.014	<0.001

Statistics: Pearson correlation test.

The best cut-off points of the hematological parameters for the diagnosis of SARS-CoV-2 infection in the patients presenting with the complaint of dyspepsia were determined by an ROC curve analysis. The optimal cut-off point predictive of SARS-CoV-2 infection was determined to be ≥ 0.045 (sensitivity: 68.4% and specificity: 85.4%, $p = 0.001$) for IG, ≥ 0.650 (sensitivity: 52.6% and specificity: 95.5%, $p = 0.001$) for IG% and ≥ 12.4 (sensitivity: 63.2% and specificity: 91.4%, $p = 0.020$) for CRP (Table 4). After we performed a risk analysis using a logistic regression model based on these cut-off points for COVID-19 diagnosis only in the patients presenting with the complaint of dyspepsia, we demonstrated that the risk increased 8.546 times ($p < 0.001$) in the patients with IG values of $\geq 0.045 \times 10^9$ L, 23.611 times ($p < 0.001$) in the patients with IG% values of ≥ 0.650, and 18.171 times ($p < 0.001$) in the patients with CRP values of ≥ 12.4 mg/L (Table 5).

Table 4. Determination of cut-off points in hematological parameters for the diagnosis of SARS-CoV-2 infection in patients presenting with dyspeptic complaints.

	Cut-Off Value	AUC	Sensitivity	Specificity	Asymptomatic 95% Confidence Interval	p
IG (10^9 L)	≥ 0.045	0.751	0.684	0.854	0.601–0.901	0.001
IG%	≥ 0.650	0.740	0.526	0.955	0.586–0.893	0.001
CRP (mg/L)	≥ 12.4	0.679	0.632	0.914	0.499–0.859	0.020

Statistics: ROC curve analysis was performed to determine the best cutoff points for GI, IG%, and CRP values to predict SARS-CoV-2 infection. Abbreviations: IG: Immature granulocyte; IG%: Immature granulocyte percentage; CRP: C-reactive protein; AUC: area under the curve.

Table 5. Risk analysis for COVID-19 diagnosis with logistic regression analysis in patients presenting with dyspeptic complaints.

	OR	95% CI	p	Risk
IG ($\geq 0.045 \times 10^9$ L)	8.546	2.854–25.596	<0.001	Present
IG% (≥ 0.650)	23.611	6.135–90.877	<0.001	Present
CRP (≥ 12.4 mg/L)	18.171	4.915–67.181	<0.001	Present

Statistics: Whether GI, G%, and CRP values pose a risk for SARS-CoV-2 infection was evaluated by logistic regression analysis. Abbreviations: IG: Immature granulocyte; IG%: Immature granulocyte percentage; CRP: C-reactive protein; OR: Odds ratio.

4. Discussion

Our study showed that COVID-19 infection may present only with resistant dyspeptic complaints in every age group. Additionally, it showed that CRP, IG, and IG% values were higher in the SARS-CoV-2-infected patient group compared to the noninfected group. These findings may guide clinicians in the early diagnosis of COVID-19 cases. SARS-CoV-2 infections have quickly spread all around the world shortly since the disease emerged in China, and a pandemic was declared by the WHO in March 2020 [2]. The main symptoms of COVID-19 were known to be coughing, fever, and shortness of breath in the beginning, but as the spread of the virus increased, the variety of symptoms began to increase, and patients have been diagnosed with COVID-19 with unexpected complaints [12]. Recent studies revealed that SARS-CoV-2 may also be spread via feces [13]. However, it was also demonstrated that SARS-CoV-2 infection may also emerge with gastrointestinal symptoms after it was determined that SARS-CoV-2 had the ability to bind to ACE2 receptors in the gastrointestinal tract [14]. The incidence of gastrointestinal symptoms in COVID-19 patients ranges from 3% to 79% [15]. Diarrhea, nausea/vomiting and weight loss are the most commonly seen gastroenterological symptoms in adult patients, while vomiting is the most common symptom reported in children. In a study of 46 COVID-19 cases with no symptoms or mild symptoms, the frequency of gastrointestinal symptoms was found to be 35%, and the frequency of dyspepsia was reported as 11% [16]. Therefore, it should be highlighted that extra care should be exercised in terms of COVID-19 when it comes to patients presenting with complaints other than respiratory symptoms [6,17].

To the best of our knowledge, our study is the only study emphasizing concurrent SARS-CoV-2 in patients presenting with the complaint of persistent dyspepsia. In our study, 19 (8%) of the 238 patients who underwent endoscopy due to persistent dyspepsia were determined to be positive for SARS-CoV-2. None of the patients who were determined to have SARS-CoV-2 had any complaints other than dyspepsia. The course of SARS-CoV-2 infection is known to be much more severe in patients with comorbidities and in geriatric patients. Although there are studies reporting that the prevalence of infection is higher in the male sex, there are also studies reporting that there is no significant correlation between SARS-CoV-2 infection and sex [18,19]. In our study, there was no statistically significant difference in terms of sex or age between the patients with and without SARS-CoV-2 infection. It was shown in a survey study, which was conducted in Japan and which included adult patients, that the COVID-19 pandemic made existing symptoms worse in 20% of patients with functional dyspepsia. It was stated in the same study that stress caused by SARS-CoV-2 was effective in worsening the existing symptoms of the patients [20]. Additionally, in a study in Italy, it was stated that functional gastrointestinal symptoms increased, especially in children and young people during the pandemic period [21]. We think that both the SARS-CoV-2 infection itself and the stress caused by COVID-19 may lead to dyspepsia or aggravate existing dyspepsia in the patients on whom we performed endoscopies. IG, IG%, and NLR values were demonstrated to increase in infectious and noninfectious inflammatory diseases, such as malignancies [22–25]. Studies have also suggested that IG% is a more predictive marker in the early diagnosis of any infection as compared to procalcitonin [26] and CRP [27] values, which are well-known markers that have been previously studied. It has been emphasized in various studies that IG% may be used in the early diagnosis of acute appendicitis, acute cholecystitis, acute pancreatitis, sepsis, and neonatal sepsis in pediatric patients [22,28–31]. Additionally, Ayres et al. [30] stated that sepsis could be ruled out in cases where the IG% value is detected as being lower than 2. In another study, Unal et al. [31] reported that IG% was an effective and inexpensive method for use in the early detection of acute necrotizing pancreatitis. None of the patients included in our study had a systemic inflammatory response (SIRS) or sepsis. In contrast to the aforementioned reports, we found that the IG and IG% levels were significantly higher in the patients with SARS-CoV-2 infection as compared to the SARS-CoV-2-negative patients.

Similarly, it was emphasized in some studies that NLR can be a useful prognostic biomarker for the detection of inflammatory diseases and sepsis [32]. Nalbant et al. [33] stated that NLR may be an independent predictive factor for the diagnosis of COVID-19 infection. However, in our study, there was no significant difference in terms of the NLR values between the SARS-CoV-2-positive and SARS-CoV-2-negative patients. This result may have occurred due to the absence of clinical symptoms and signs suggesting sepsis and/or inflammatory disease other than dyspepsia or early-stage COVID-19 in the patients we included in our study. Van der Geest et al. [34] reported that IG% and CRP may be interchangeable, while combining CRP and IG% findings provides better results for predicting microbial infection. In our study, the CRP values were determined to be significantly higher in the SARS-CoV-2-positive patients in comparison to the SARS-CoV-2-negative patients. There were significant positive correlations between the CRP values and the IG and IG% values (r: 0.279, p: 0.014; r: 0.892 $p < 0.001$, respectively).

Ha et al. [35] determined an IG% cut-off point of 0.5 for the differentiation of complicated and uncomplicated sepsis. In another study, the cut-off point for IG% was determined to be 0.4 (sensitivity: 69.8% and specificity: 29.5%) in predicting sepsis based on clinical diagnosis [28]. There is no diagnostic study in the literature which was conducted with IG and IG% to predict SARS-CoV-2 infection in patients presenting only with the complaint of dyspepsia. Therefore, we determined the optimal cut-off points for CRP, IG, and IG% with an ROC curve analysis to predict SARS-CoV-2 infection in our study. Additionally, in contrast with the literature, we performed a risk analysis for SARS-CoV-2 infection using logistic regression analysis according to these cut-off points.

Limitations

Our study included both pediatric and adult patients. Another strength of our study is that it is the first study to develop an early diagnostic marker of COVID-19 infection in patients with dyspepsia using frequently used hematological data. The retrospective nature of the study, the low number of pediatric patients, and the low number of patients with COVID-19 infection were the limitations of our study.

5. Conclusions

It should be noted that dyspepsia may also be a symptom in SARS-CoV-2 infected patients. In this period when the world cannot completely rid itself of the COVID-19 pandemic, our study showed that dyspepsia, a nonspecific complaint for COVID-19, can be suspected and diagnosed early with simple hematological data, such as immature granulocyte percentages and counts. However, these findings need to be supported by larger and more comprehensive studies.

Author Contributions: Data curation, S.G. and M.I.; Formal analysis, B.K.; Investigation, K.G.; Methodology, K.G.; Resources, K.G.; Supervision, K.G. and S.G.; Writing—original draft, M.I.; Writing—review and editing, K.G., S.G. and B.K. All authors have read and agreed to the published version of the manuscript.

Funding: This research received no external funding.

Institutional Review Board Statement: The study was conducted in accordance with the Declaration of Helsinki and was approved by the local ethics committee of Sutcu Imam University, Kahramanmaras, Turkey (decision date: 25 January 2021, session: 2021/04, no. 10).

Informed Consent Statement: Patient consent was waived due to the retrospective design of this study.

Data Availability Statement: The datasets used and/or analysed during the current study are available from the corresponding author on reasonable request.

Conflicts of Interest: The authors declare that they have no conflict of interest.

References

1. Ma, C.; Cong, Y.; Zhang, H. COVID-19 and the Digestive System. *Am. J. Gastroenterol.* **2020**, *115*, 1003–1006. [CrossRef] [PubMed]
2. World Health Organization. WHO Director-General's Opening Remarks at the Media Briefing on COVID-19–11 March 2020. Available online: https://www.who.int/director-general/speeches/detail/who-director-general-s-opening-remarks-at-the-media-briefing-on-covid-19---11-march-2020 (accessed on 15 February 2022).
3. Lazar, M.; Barbu, E.C.; Chitu, C.E.; Anghel, A.M.J.; Niculae, C.M.; Manea, E.D.; Damalan, A.C.; Bel, A.A.; Patrascu, R.R.; Hristea, A.; et al. Pericardial Involvement in Severe COVID-19 Patients. *Medicina* **2022**, *58*, 1093. [CrossRef]
4. Orlandi, M.; Landini, N.; Sambataro, G.; Nardi, C.; Tofani, L.; Bruni, C.; Bellando-Randone, S.; Blagojevic, J.; Melchiorre, D.; Hughes, M.; et al. The role of chest CT in deciphering interstitial lung involvement: Systemic sclerosis versus COVID-19. *Rheumatology* **2022**, *61*, 1600–1609. [CrossRef] [PubMed]
5. Dong, Z.Y.; Xiang, B.J.; Jiang, M.; Sun, M.J.; Dai, C. The Prevalence of Gastrointestinal Symptoms, Abnormal Liver Function, Digestive System Disease and Liver Disease in COVID-19 Infection: A Systematic Review and Meta-Analysis. *J. Clin. Gastroenterol.* **2021**, *55*, 67–76. [CrossRef] [PubMed]
6. Silva, F.A.F.D.; Brito, B.B.; Santos, M.L.C.; Marques, H.S.; Silva, R.T.D., Jr.; Carvalho, L.S.; Vieira, E.S.; Oliveira, M.V.; de Melo, F.F. COVID-19 gastrointestinal manifestations: A systematic review. *Rev. Soc. Bras. Med. Trop.* **2020**, *53*, e20200714. [CrossRef] [PubMed]
7. Oshima, T.; Fukui, H.; Watari, J.; Miwa, H. Childhood abuse history is associated with the development of dyspepsia: A population-based survey in Japan. *J. Gastroenterol.* **2015**, *50*, 744–750. [CrossRef]

8. Moayyedi, P.; Lacy, B.E.; Andrews, C.N.; Enns, R.A.; Howden, C.W.; Vakil, N. ACG and CAG Clinical Guideline: Management of Dyspepsia. *J. Gastroenterol.* **2017**, *112*, 988–1013. [CrossRef]
9. Ansari-Lari, M.A.; Kickler, T.S.; Borowitz, M.J. Immature granulocyte measurement using the Sysmex XE-2100. Relationship to infection and sepsis. *Am. J. Clin. Pathol.* **2003**, *120*, 795–799. [CrossRef] [PubMed]
10. Park, J.H.; Byeon, H.J.; Lee, K.H.; Lee, J.W.; Kronbichler, A.; Eisenhut, M.; Shin, J.I. Delta neutrophil index (DNI) as a novel diagnostic and prognostic marker of infection: A systematic review and meta-analysis. *Inflamm. Res.* **2017**, *66*, 863–870. [CrossRef] [PubMed]
11. Tarik, A.; Soukaina, R.; Samir, M.; Asmae, S.; Ahlame, B.; Rida, B.; Yasser, A.; Ilham, E.; Noureddine, E.; Hassan, S.; et al. Gastrointestinal manifestations during COVID-19 virus infection: A Moroccan prospective study. *Arab. J. Gastroenterol.* **2021**, *22*, 305–309. [CrossRef]
12. ISARIC Clinical Characterisation Group. COVID-19 symptoms at hospital admission vary with age and sex: Results from the ISARIC prospective multinational observational study. *Infection* **2021**, *49*, 889–905. [CrossRef] [PubMed]
13. Holshue, M.L.; DeBolt, C.; Lindquist, S.; Lofy, K.H.; Wiesman, J.; Bruce, H.; Spitters, C.; Ericson, K.; Wilkerson, S.; Tural, A.; et al. Washington State 2019-nCoV Case Investigation Team. First Case of 2019 Novel Coronavirus in the United States. *N. Engl. J. Med.* **2020**, *382*, 929–936. [CrossRef] [PubMed]
14. Jin, X.; Lian, J.S.; Hu, J.H.; Gao, J.; Zheng, L.; Zhang, Y.M.; Hao, S.R.; Jia, H.Y.; Cai, H.; Zhang, X.L.; et al. Epidemiological, clinical and virological characteristics of 74 cases of coronavirus-infected disease 2019 (COVID-19) with gastrointestinal symptoms. *Gut* **2020**, *69*, 1002–1009. [CrossRef]
15. Tian, Y.; Rong, L.; Nian, W.; He, Y. Review article: Gastrointestinal features in COVID-19 and the possibility of faecal transmission. *Aliment. Pharmacol. Ther.* **2020**, *51*, 843–851. [CrossRef]
16. Park, S.K.; Lee, C.W.; Park, D.I.; Woo, H.Y.; Cheong, H.S.; Shin, H.C.; Ahn, K.; Kwon, M.J.; Joo, E.J. Detection of SARS-CoV-2 in Fecal Samples From Patients With Asymptomatic and Mild COVID-19 in Korea. *Clin. Gastroenterol Hepatol.* **2021**, *19*, 1387–1394. [CrossRef] [PubMed]
17. Fang, D.; Ma, J.; Guan, J.; Wang, M.; Song, Y.; Tian, D.; Li, P. Manifestations of digestive system in hospitalized patients with novel coronavirus pneumonia in Wuhan, China: A single-center, descriptive study. *Chin. J. Dig.* **2020**, *40*, E005. [CrossRef]
18. Wenham, C.; Smith, J.; Morgan, R. Gender and COVID-19 Working Group. COVID-19: The gendered impacts of the outbreak. *Lancet* **2020**, *395*, 846–848. [CrossRef]
19. Jin, J.M.; Bai, P.; He, W.; Wu, F.; Liu, X.F.; Han, D.M.; Liu, S.; Yang, J.K. Gender Differences in Patients With COVID-19: Focus on Severity and Mortality. *Front. Public Health* **2020**, *8*, 152. [CrossRef] [PubMed]
20. Oshima, T.; Siah, K.T.H.; Yoshimoto, T.; Miura, K.; Tomita, T.; Fukui, H.; Miwa, H. Impacts of the COVID-19 pandemic on functional dyspepsia and irritable bowel syndrome: A population-based survey. *J. Gastroenterol. Hepatol.* **2021**, *36*, 1820–1827. [CrossRef] [PubMed]
21. Farello, G.; Di Lucia, A.; Fioravanti, B.; Tambucci, R.; Stagi, S.; Gaudino, R. Analysis of the impact of COVID-19 pandemic on functional gastrointestinal disorders among paediatric population. *Eur. Rev. Med. Pharmacol. Sci.* **2021**, *25*, 5836–5842. [CrossRef] [PubMed]
22. Kim, T.Y.; Kim, S.J.; Kim, Y.S.; Lee, J.W.; Park, E.J.; Lee, S.J.; Lee, K.J.; Cha, Y.S. Delta neutrophil index as an early predictive marker of severe acute pancreatitis in the emergency department. *Unit. Eur. Gastroenterol. J.* **2019**, *7*, 488–495. [CrossRef] [PubMed]
23. Celik, I.H.; Arifoglu, I.; Arslan, Z.; Aksu, G.; Bas, A.Y.; Demirel, N. The value of delta neutrophil index in neonatal sepsis diagnosis, follow-up and mortality prediction. *Early Hum. Dev.* **2019**, *131*, 6–9. [CrossRef] [PubMed]
24. Bozan, M.B.; Yazar, F.M.; Kale, İ.T.; Yüzbaşıoğlu, M.F.; Boran, Ö.F.; Bozan, A.A. Delta Neutrophil Index and Neutrophil-to-Lymphocyte Ratio in the Differentiation of Thyroid Malignancy and Nodular Goiter. *World J. Surg.* **2021**, *45*, 507–514. [CrossRef] [PubMed]
25. Barut, O.; Demirkol, M.K.; Kucukdurmaz, F.; Sahinkanat, T.; Resim, S. Pre-treatment Delta Neutrophil Index as a Predictive Factor in Renal Cell Carcinoma. *J. Coll. Phys. Surg. Pak.* **2021**, *31*, 156–161. [CrossRef]
26. Wacker, C.; Prkno, A.; Brunkhorst, F.M.; Schlattmann, P. Procalcitonin as a diagnostic marker for sepsis: A systematic review and meta-analysis. *Lancet Infect. Dis.* **2013**, *13*, 426–435. [CrossRef]
27. Povoa, P. C-reactive protein: A valuable marker of sepsis. *Intens. Care Med.* **2002**, *28*, 235–243. [CrossRef] [PubMed]
28. Shin, D.H.; Cho, Y.S.; Cho, G.C.; Ahn, H.C.; Park, S.M.; Lim, S.W.; Oh, Y.T.; Cho, J.W.; Park, S.O.; Lee, Y.H. Delta neutrophil index as an early predictor of acute appendicitis and acute complicated appendicitis in adults. *World J. Emerg. Surg.* **2017**, *12*, 32. [CrossRef] [PubMed]
29. Lee, S.J.; Park, E.J.; Lee, K.J.; Cha, Y.S. The delta neutrophil index is an early predictive marker of severe acute cholecystitis. *Dig. Liver Dis.* **2019**, *51*, 1593–1598. [CrossRef]
30. Ayres, L.S.; Sgnaolin, V.; Munhoz, T.P. Immature granulocytes index as early marker of sepsis. *Int. J. Lab. Hematol.* **2019**, *41*, 392–396. [CrossRef] [PubMed]
31. Ünal, Y.; Barlas, A.M. Role of increased immature granulocyte percentage in the early prediction of acute necrotizing pancreatitis. *Turk. J. Trauma Emerg. Surg.* **2019**, *25*, 177–182. [CrossRef]
32. Huang, Z.; Fu, Z.; Huang, W.; Huang, K. Prognostic value of neutrophil-to-lymphocyte ratio in sepsis: A meta-analysis. *Am. J. Emerg. Med.* **2020**, *38*, 641–647. [CrossRef] [PubMed]

33. Nalbant, A.; Kaya, T.; Varim, C.; Yaylaci, S.; Tamer, A.; Cinemre, H. Can the neutrophil/lymphocyte ratio (NLR) have a role in the diagnosis of coronavirus 2019 disease (COVID-19)? *Rev. Assoc. Med. Bras.* **2020**, *66*, 746–751. [CrossRef] [PubMed]
34. Van der Geest, P.J.; Mohseni, M.; Brouwer, R.; van der Hoven, B.; Steyerberg, E.W.; Groeneveld, A.B. Immature granulocytes predict microbial infection and its adverse sequelae in the intensive care unit. *J. Crit. Care.* **2014**, *29*, 523–527. [CrossRef] [PubMed]
35. Ha, S.O.; Park, S.H.; Park, S.H.; Park, J.S.; Huh, J.W.; Lim, C.M.; Koh, Y.; Hong, S.B.; Jang, S. Fraction of immature granulocytes reflects severity but not mortality in sepsis. *Scand. J. Clin. Lab. Invest.* **2015**, *75*, 36–43. [CrossRef] [PubMed]

Small Bowel Diverticulosis and COVID-19: Awareness Is the Key: A Case Series and Review of the Literature

Petros Bangeas [1,2,*], Nikolaos Konstantinidis [1], Tania Chrisopoulou [2], Despoina Karatzia [1], Alexandros Giakoustidis [1] and Vasileios N. Papadopoulos [1]

1. 1st University Surgery Department, Papageorgiou Hospital, Aristotle University of Thessaloniki, 54124 Thessaloniki, Greece; nikos4kanti@yahoo.gr (N.K.); despoinakaratzia@hotmail.com (D.K.); alexgiakoustidis@gmail.com (A.G.); papadvas@auth.gr (V.N.P.)
2. Department of Radiology, Genesis General Clinic, 54301 Thessaloniki, Greece; chrysopouloutania@gmail.com
* Correspondence: pbangeas@gmail.com

Abstract: Small bowel non-Meckelian diverticulosis is a rare condition with only a few published cases despite being described over 200 years ago. In the midst of the COVID-19 pandemic, studies suggested that many patients may experience gastrointestinal manifestations. Intestinal symptoms could worsen the inflammation and infection associated with small bowel diverticulitis. Here we present three cases: one with inflammation and rupture in a COVID-19 patient and another as an asymptomatic detection. The third case involved recurrence after the first laparoscopic lavage approach. Furthermore, we provide a mini-review of the literature to emphasize the importance of considering this entity in the differential diagnosis of an acute abdomen. In the majority of cases involving small bowel diverticula, conservative management is the preferred approach. However, when complications arise, surgical intervention, including enteroctomy and primary anastomosis, may be necessary to achieve optimal outcomes.

Keywords: small bowel non-Meckelian; diverticulitis; COVID-19

1. Introduction

Small bowel non-Meckelian (SBNMD) diverticulosis is an uncommon disorder with a prevalence ranging from 0.06% to 4% [1–4]. While diverticula are more commonly found in the colon, they can also occur in the small bowel. It typically occurs in the sixth and seventh decades of life, with a significant majority of 80% being over 40 years old at the time of the diagnosis [4]. Multiple jejunal diverticula, especially in the proximal site, are detected in 80% of cases. The remaining 15% of diverticula are located in the ileum, while the remaining 5% occur in both the jejunum and ileum [5]. Both are usually smaller in size, multiple, and isolated. Meckelian diverticula are congenital abnormalities of the small intestine, but non-Meckelian diverticulitis is not associated with this congenital anomaly [1]. From a pathological point of view, SBNMD are deemed "false", in contrast to Meckel's diverticula located on the anti-mesenteric site [1,2]. The wide range of atypical symptoms, such as vague abdominal pain, flatulence, diarrhea, and melaena, in combination with its rare occurrence, can lead to a delayed diagnosis and extreme mortality rates [6,7]. Various imaging modalities can be utilized to aid in the diagnosis of non-Meckelian small bowel diverticulitis. A computed tomography (CT) scan is typically the first-line imaging modality used to evaluate patients with suspected diverticulitis. CT can identify inflamed or perforated diverticula, as well as complications such as abscess formation or bowel obstruction. Magnetic resonance imaging (MRI) may also be used to evaluate non-Meckelian small bowel diverticulitis, particularly in cases where radiation exposure is a concern [4–7]. In addition to CT and MRI, other imaging modalities such as small bowel follow-through studies or enteroclysis may be utilized to evaluate the extent of diverticulitis and any associated complications. Endoscopic retrograde cholangiopancreatography (ERCP) may also be performed to visualize the small bowel and assess for the presence of diverticula especially in case of duodenum localization [2–5].

Complications frequently occur with colonic diverticula, which are commonly described. These complications include inflammation, perforation, bleeding, and obstruction. The primary diagnostic tool that we use is abdominal computed tomography (CT) [4].

The pandemic has had a significant impact on the management of diverticulitis cases, with delays in seeking medical attention leading to more severe cases upon presentation to healthcare facilities. This delay can be attributed to various factors, including fear of contracting COVID-19 in a healthcare setting, limited access to medical resources due to the overwhelming burden on hospitals, and the reluctance of individuals to seek medical care for what they perceive as non-emergent conditions. Additionally, the strain on healthcare systems has resulted in the postponement or cancellation of non-urgent elective procedures, including colonoscopies, which are crucial in the diagnosis and management of diverticulitis. As a result, many cases of diverticulitis may have gone undiagnosed or untreated, leading to an increased risk of rupture and its associated complications [4–6].

Recent studies have suggested a potential link between colitis, diverticulitis, and COVID-19, indicating that individuals with inflammatory bowel diseases may be at an increased risk of experiencing more severe symptoms and complications if they contract the virus. The reasoning behind this correlation lies in the role of the immune system. Colitis is known to weaken the immune system and predispose individuals to infections. When faced with the SARS-CoV-2 virus, individuals with colitis may struggle to mount an effective immune response, leading to a heightened risk of severe illness and complications associated with COVID-19. Furthermore, patients with colitis often require immunosuppressive medications to manage their condition, which could further compromise their ability to fight off the virus. This highlights the importance of careful management and monitoring of individuals with colitis during the ongoing COVID-19 pandemic. It is crucial for healthcare providers to recognize the potential correlation between inflammatory bowel diseases and COVID-19 and take appropriate measures to protect and support individuals with colitis, such as prioritizing vaccination, closely monitoring symptoms, and providing timely medical intervention when necessary [5–7].

The fact is that the exact mechanism has not been determined; however, it appears that the SARS-CoV-2 virus (COVID-19) primarily targets the respiratory tract through its affinity for ACE2 receptors. These receptors are also prevalent in intestinal cells, leading to symptoms affecting both the respiratory and gastrointestinal systems. COVID-19 affects the bloodstream, causing hyperactivity in platelets and cytokine storms. This can result in damage to the gut barrier and changes to the gut microbiota. Additionally, intestinal vessel thrombosis can occur, leading to malabsorption and malnutrition. These negative effects can increase the severity of the disease and have both short- and long-term consequences, including gut inflammation and worsening of inflammatory bowel diseases [8,9]. All these had a significant impact on the management of diverticulitis, leading to an increased risk of rupture and potentially life-threatening outcomes. It is crucial for individuals to seek prompt medical attention for symptoms of diverticulitis and for healthcare systems to prioritize the management of these cases to prevent severe complications.

Management of SBNMD typically includes a combination of conservative and surgical interventions. The specific treatment approach depends on the rupture's severity, complications, and the patient's overall condition. Every stable patient with localized inflammation and without any radiologic sign of perforation is treated conservatively with bowel rest and broad-spectrum IV antibiotics. If the patient does not show clinical improvement within 48–72 h or if generalized peritonitis or perforation is detected, an exploratory laparotomy may be necessary, which involves small bowel resection with anastomosis [5–7].

Herein, we present three cases of SBNMD. The first case involved a COVID-19-positive patient with rupture, while the second case was discovered incidentally. The third case involved recurrence after the first laparoscopic lavage approach. The cases discussed in this report highlight the need for careful management and monitoring of SBNMD, particularly in high-risk patients such as those with COVID-19. Additionally, these cases underscore the importance of prompt detection and intervention in cases of recurrence. It is hoped that this report will contribute to the existing body of knowledge regarding the diagnosis and treatment of SBNMD and, ultimately, lead to better outcomes for patients afflicted with this condition. In addition, a review with a statistical analysis of all the cases reported in the past literature, discussing the most common clinical features, was performed. Also, we proposed the role of laparoscopic surgery as a therapeutic option in disease management.

2. Materials and Methods

A literature review was performed using PubMed, Scopus, and Science Direct. The search terms employed were "small bowel diverticulosis", "jejunal diverticulitis", and "Ileus diverticulitis". Since 2010, 352 articles have been published.

Among these, 217 well-documented papers were identified. There were no restrictions on the ages of the articles included in this review. One hundred eighty-six articles were in English, while 31 were in other languages. All these studies were carefully studied. We had only full texts, case reports, and case series articles in the final assessment. We finally selected 38 articles (41 patients), and a database with the patients' characteristics was created and is shown in the Prisma chart below (Scheme 1).

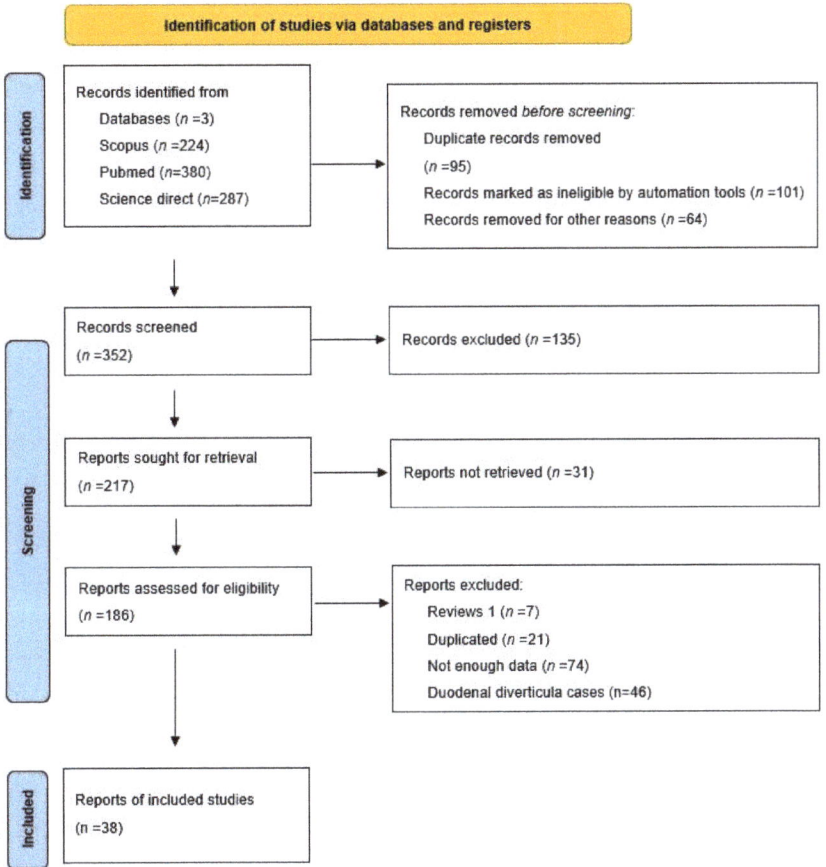

Scheme 1. Prisma chart with studies included in our manuscript.

The database included sex, age, diverticula location, symptoms, diagnostic methods, treatment management, and complications. The cases that fulfilled all these seven criteria were included in the statistical analysis. Three additional cases were added from the clinical experience of the authors of this article. Thus, a total of 44 patients were included in the statistical analysis. After obtaining ethical approval and participant consent, personal data were removed, and all clinical data were collected. In order to ensure that our study was conducted with the utmost respect for ethical guidelines and research standards, it was crucial to prepare a CARE checklist (Appendix A). Descriptive statistics were used to express the results appropriately. Means, medians, and SDs were used for continuous variables and frequencies for categorical variables. The statistical significance was set at $p < 0.05$. The statistical analysis was performed using SPSS version 25 (SPSS Inc., Chicago, IL, USA).

3. Case Report

3.1. Case 1

A 45-year-old male presented to our emergency department, complaining about abdominal pain, particularly on the left side, that had been ongoing for 48 h. The clinical examination revealed abdominal distension and tenderness. The laboratory results showed a mildly elevated white blood cell count (9.93×10^9/L) and neutrophilia (88%). During the preoperative examination, it was discovered incidentally that the patient had contracted COVID-19 infection. An emergency CT scan of the abdomen revealed free air, fluid collection in the left abdomen, and two small bowel diverticula in the jejunum with local phlegm (Figure 1a). From the patient's past medical history, there is no record of diverticula except experiencing upper gastrointestinal bleeding 11 years ago. Additionally, the patient had a history of cardiac arrest and a pacemaker implanted 15 years prior.

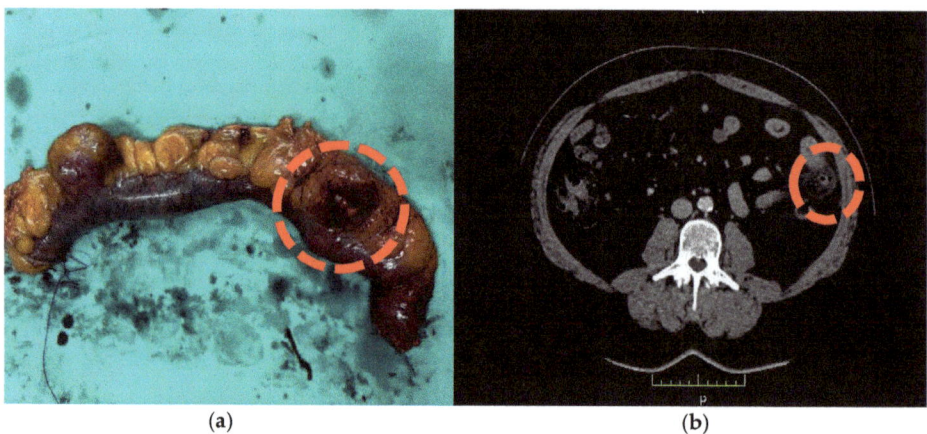

Figure 1. (**a**) Case 1 ruptured jejunum diverticula. (**b**) Abdominal CT, showing ruptured non-Meckelian diverticula. In Circle we can see the intraoperative (**a**) and radiological imaging (**b**) ruptured part of diverticula.

Informed written consent was obtained from the patient, and he was taken to the operating theater for an exploratory laparoscopy, where a ruptured part of the jejunum was found (Figure 1b). A partial small bowel laparoscopic enterectomy was carried out with primary side-to-side intracorporeal anastomosis with an endoscopic linear stapler and PDS 2-0 running suture. The patient was discharged from the surgery without drainages and received clear fluids in the afternoon after the surgery. He was mobilized six hours after surgery. Throughout the hospitalization period, he remained stable, and on the third postoperative day, he was discharged. The patient followed a fast-track post-operative protocol (ERAS), which included mobile communication and visits from a specialist nurse.

3.2. Case 2

A 75-year-old male presented to our department due to a rectal tumor of 9 cm from the anal verge. The patient underwent an operating theater for a scheduled low anterior resection. During the operation, multiple jejunal diverticula were identified (Figure 2b). Upon further examination, it was determined that these diverticula were not inflamed, therefore obviating the necessity for their removal. It is worth noting that no diverticula were mentioned in the preoperative CT of the abdomen.

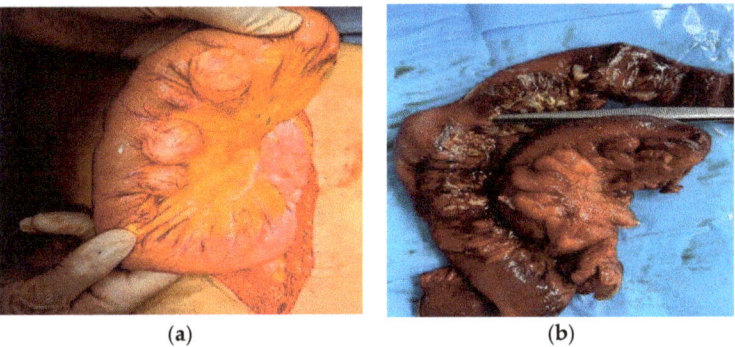

Figure 2. (a) Incidentally identified SBNM diverticula. (b) A ruptured ileum diverticula with inflammation extension in sigmoid colon.

3.3. Case 3

Upon presentation, a patient aged 46 years complained of acute abdominal pain, which had persisted for a period of 24 h. The clinical examination revealed abdominal distension and tenderness. The laboratory results indicated an elevated white blood cell count of $16.93 \times 10^9/L$ and neutrophilia of 90%. During a preoperative examination, it was incidentally discovered that the patient had contracted COVID-19. Subsequently, an emergency computed tomography (CT) scan of the abdomen revealed the presence of free air, fluid collection in the left abdomen, and diverticula in the sigmoid colon with local phlegm (as depicted in Figure 1a). The patient had no significant medical history prior to this incident. In order to investigate the condition further, the patient underwent an investigative laparoscopy in the operating theater. During the procedure, it was observed that there was no presence of fecal content. However, a purulent collection was identified and subsequently drained. Further investigation revealed a small rupture in the ileum diverticula, which was repaired using laparoscopic suturing. It is noteworthy that the rupture was not found in the sigmoid colon. This was followed by laparoscopic lavage and drains placement. The postoperative theater was uneventful. Following surgical intervention, the patient in question received a regimen of antibiotics, specifically meropenem and metronidazole. Despite this treatment, on the third day post-surgery, the patient presented with a fever of 39.1 °C and leukocytosis ($27 \times 10^9/L$). Consequently, an exploratory laparoscopy procedure was conducted, ultimately exposing a substantial intra-abdominal collection. Following laparoscopic lavage, we determined that the inflamed section of the ileum required an enterectomy and side-to-side anastomosis. Furthermore, the inflammation had significantly corroded the walls of the sigmoid colon, necessitating a partial sigmoidectomy with a hand-sewn end-to-end anastomosis (Figure 2b). The patient was administered clear fluids on the first postoperative day and was mobilized just twelve hours after surgery. Throughout their hospitalization, the patient remained stable and was discharged on the fifth postoperative day after the second surgery.

4. Results

After conducting a literature review, we determined the characteristics of jejunal diverticula based on various factors, including sex, age, length, location of the diverticula, significant symptoms, type of procedure, survival rates, and potential complications categorized by Clavien–Dindo classification [2,4–7,10–44].

Regarding sex, 63.63% were male (28 patients), whereas 36.37% were female (16 patients). The ratio between males and females was 2:1, suggesting a male predominance in the reported population. Our database is shown below (Table 1).

Table 1. Diverticula cases publication.

Year	Author	Disease Location	Cases	Age/Gender	Treatment
2017	Marcano	Jejunal	1	71/male	Conservative
2019	Almaki	Jejunal	1	65/Male	Open Surgery
2019	Aispuro	Jejunal	1	86/Male	Open Surgery
2019	Saritas	Jejunal	2	36/Female	Open surgery
		Ileus		75/Female	Open surgery
2020	Ghandour	Jejunal	3	71/Male	Open Surgery
		Jejunal		69/Male	Open Surgery
		Jejunal		55/Male	Conservative
2020	Kunishi	Jejunal	1	41/Male	Conservative
2020	Leigh	Jejunal	1	59/Male	Open Surgery
2020	Ramzee	Jejunal	1	69/Male	Open Surgery
2020	Sammartino	Jejunal	1	91/Male	Open Surgery
2020	Yeung	Jejunal	1	83/Male	Open Surgery
2021	Alyekbeni	Jejunal	1	70/Male	Conservative
2021	Anjum	Jejunal	1	70/Male	Open Surgery
2021	Chung	Jejunal	1	69/Female	Open Surgery
2021	Duggan	Jejunal	1	78/Male	Open Surgery
2021	Giufrida	Jejunal	1	54/Female	Open Surgery
2021	Hardon	Jejunal	1	37/Female	Open Surgery
2021	Khsiba	Jejunal	1	76/Female	Conservative
2021	Kim	Jejunal	1	65/Female	Conservative
2021	Mendo	Ileus	1	73/Male	Open Surgery
2021	Rajaguru	Ileus	1	74/Male	Open Surgery
2021	Vayzband	Jejunal	1	71/Male	Open Surgery
2021	Watanabe	Distal Jejunal	1	72/Male	Open Surgery
2022	Abdelohamil	Jejunal	1	69/Female	Open Surgery
2022	Beti	Jejunal	1	83/Male	Open Surgery
2022	Coelen	Jejunal	1	85/Male	Open Surgery
2022	Eifanagely	Jejunal	1	79/Female	Conservative
2022	Glasser	Ileus	1	57/Male	Open Surgery
2022	Imasato	Jejunal	1	76/Female	Open Surgery
2022	Karna	Jejunal	1	89/Female	Embolization
2022	Lutaya	Jejunal	1	89/Female	Open Surgery
2022	Massoir	Jejunal	1	84/Female	Open Surgery
2022	Matli	Jejunal	1	41/Male	Conservative
2022	Scheesee	Jejunal	1	85/Male	Open Surgery
2022	Pajtak	Jejunal	1	88/Female	Open Surgery
2022	Prough	Jejunal	1	65/Male	Open Surgery
2022	Waiter	Ileus	1	59/Male	Open Surgery

Based on our database (Table 1), it appears that diverticula are typically found in the jejunum, as illustrated in Figure 3 (31 patients, 70.45%), with only 9 patients with diverticula found in the proximal ileus (20.45%) and 4 patients with diverticula in the distal ileus (9.09%).

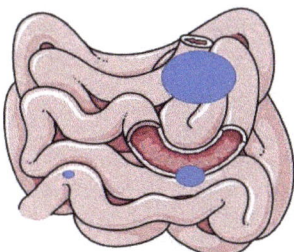

Figure 3. SMNMD localization.

The age distribution is shown in Figure 4, from which it is concluded that jejunum diverticula most frequently appeared in the age ranges of 64–72, 73–81, and 82–91 years. The median age of the 44 cases (100%) was 71 ± 14.40 years, ranging from 36 to 91 years. The distribution of age among male and female patients was compared, and it was found that the age at which the tumor appeared did not differ statistically between males and females (70.12 ± 13.27 and 70 ± 15.99 years, respectively; $p = 0.98$).

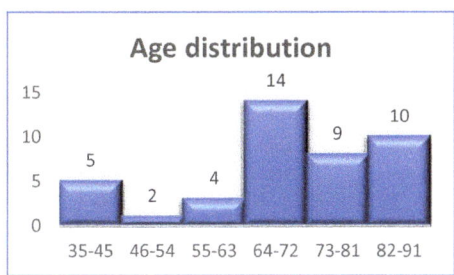

Figure 4. Age distribution.

The symptoms of SBNMD were also evaluated and are shown in Figure 5. Symptoms were characterized as inflammatory without rupture (1) (16 patients, 36.36%), perforation (2) (19 patients, 43.18%), bleeding (3) (1 patient, 2.27%), (4) obstruction (6 patients, 13.63%), and non-specific/random (5) (2 patients, 4.54%).

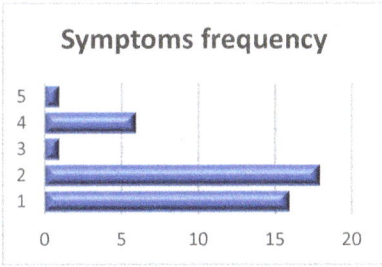

Figure 5. Diverticula symptoms.

Out of 44 patients, only 8 (18.18%) received conservative treatment, while the majority (35 patients, 79.54%) required surgical intervention. Diverticula were discovered accidentally in two patients (4.54%) without signs of inflammation, and no interventions were performed. Of the 44 patients under study, open laparotomy was performed on 33 (75.01%) patients. Conversely, laparoscopic surgery was conducted on only three (6.81%) patients, while the remaining eight patients (18.18%) received conservative care. This indicated that the majority of patients preferred open laparotomy over the laparoscopic approach. The findings underscore the need for further investigation to determine the factors that contribute to patient preferences for open laparotomy and whether laparoscopic surgery is a viable alternative for patients undergoing the procedure.

The median hospitalization was 7 ± 2.37 days, ranging from 3 to 16 days, depending on the treatment option. Hospitalization periods were found to be prolonged for patients who underwent open surgery or were treated using conservative methods.

In order to standardize the complications of our study we use Clavien–Dindo classification, which is a widely used system to categorize surgical complications based on their severity and the treatment required to address them. In accordance with the utilized classification system, it was determined that a total of 29 patients (65.90%) did not necessitate pharmacological, surgical, endoscopic, or radiological interventions (Clavien–Dindo I). Conversely, 12 patients (27.27%) received antibiotic care and parental nutrition (Clavien–Dindo II). Further, two patients (4.54%) required additional surgical procedures (Clavien–Dindo IIIb), while regrettably, a single patient (2.27%) succumbed to their illness during the post-operative period (Clavien–Dindo V).

5. Discussion

Jejuno-ileal diverticulitis, a condition involving inflammation of the diverticula in the small intestine, was initially identified by Sommering in 1794 and further researched by Sir Astley Cooper in 1804 [1]. Due to its low prevalence, there have been only a few reported cases since then. The pathophysiology still needs to be fully understood. These are false diverticula of the small intestine, similar to colonic diverticula, where the mucosa and submucosa protrude through the muscular wall. We assume that an elevated intraluminal pressure combined with bowel wall weakness causes these cases. While they are usually asymptomatic, they can lead to life-threatening outcomes when complicated [2,5,8,11].

In the case of uncomplicated SBNMDs, no specific symptoms can lead to the diagnosis. These patients usually complain of abdominal pain, which sometimes radiates in the back, nausea, emesis, fever, and constipation. Due to the greater frequency in the older adult population, where many other health issues or previous surgical history can co-exist, the diagnosis could be challenging [2,5,7,27–34].

Numerous reports have emerged during the COVID-19 period regarding inflammation and bowel ruptures. This is a matter of concern, and we should examine these reports closely to determine the root cause of such incidents and identify measures to mitigate them in the future. Several scientific investigations have highlighted a decline in the number of visits related to diverticular disease during the COVID-19 pandemic. The reduction in visits can be attributed to various factors, including the implementation of social distancing measures, fear of contracting the virus, and limited access to healthcare facilities. However, despite the decrease in overall visits, there has been a significant increase in the prevalence of severe cases. This trend is likely due to a delay in presentation as patients may be reluctant to seek medical attention due to concerns about exposure to the virus. Additionally, there are still instances of COVID-19 patients experiencing a worsening of their diverticular disease, which may be attributed to the effect of the virus on the immune system. Therefore, it is crucial to raise awareness about the risks of delaying medical care and to encourage patients to seek timely treatment to avoid potentially life-threatening complications [35–37].

In some studies, it seems that gut enterocytes have been determined to be significant targets of the COVID-19 virus. The virus can enter the cells of the ileum, colon, and esophagus by using Angiotensin-converting enzyme 2 receptors and transmembrane serine protease 2 (TMPRSS2) as a mediator [8,9]. This can lead to gut inflammation and exacerbation of inflammatory bowel diseases, causing negative effects that can worsen the disease severity in both the short and the long term [9].

A comprehensive patient history must be obtained to rule out other conditions such as appendicitis, cholecystitis, colonic diverticulitis, pancreatitis, bowel obstruction, or foreign body perforation [3,4,8–20,24,34]. An abdominal X-ray can help detect perforation or obstruction but cannot establish a diagnosis on its own. The surgeon must maintain a heightened level of suspicion to ensure the procedure's accuracy and safety. This involves being vigilant and attentive to any potential risks or complications that may arise during the surgery.

Currently, the gold standard imaging study for abdominal scans still involves using CT scans with both oral and intravenous contrast. Due to the rarity of the disease, there are instances in the literature where the diagnosis was not clearly established before the exploratory intervention but only during exploratory laparoscopy. In our cases, the preoperative CT scan was exact for the site and the number of the ill-defined diverticula [28–44].

As mentioned before, inflammation is the most common complication, followed by perforation. First-line treatment for uncomplicated cases involves IV antibiotics and bowel rest strategies. An annual monitoring protocol, including a clinical examination and CT scan of the abdomen, is necessary in case of accidental detection. Prior history-based clinical suspicion is also important [4,28,35,44–49].

Surgical intervention must be undertaken without delay in cases of sepsis, instability, or severe comorbidities following perforation. These complications could be severe and lead to serious difficulties if not addressed promptly. The type of procedure (open or laparoscopic) does not seem to play an important role and appears to be determined by the surgeon's preference and center experience. If a patient has a good performance status, surgeons could perform an exploratory laparoscopy and proceed with a conversion procedure (laparotomy) if needed. The length of the bowel resection is also a matter of discussion. There are cases in the literature where the extreme length of bowel disease does not make wide resection feasible [40,47–51]. Most surgeons resect only the complicated diverticular disease and leave the uncomplicated diverticula behind. Based on summarized publications, we create an algorithm in order to manage jejunum diverticulum (Figure 6).

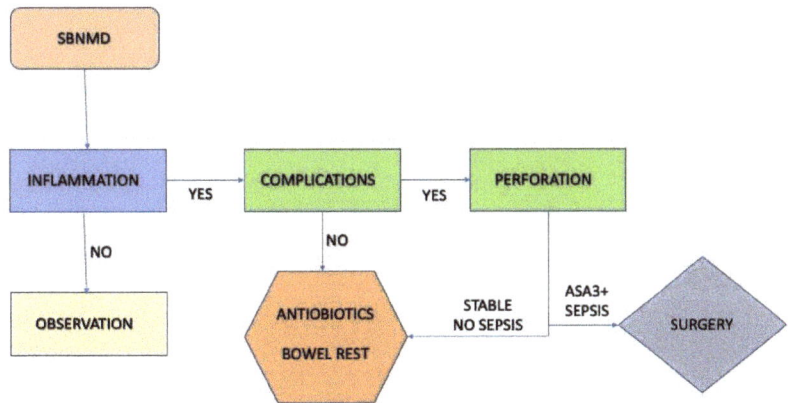

Figure 6. Suggested strategy of SBNMD treatment.

According to our algorithm, in the first case, the patient was hemodynamically stable but had comorbidities (ASA3). The CT scan revealed free abdominal air caused by the perforation of one of two jejunal diverticula. The decision was made to perform surgery on the patient without delay. An exploratory laparoscopy was our first choice, while laparoscopic lavage is seen as an acceptable and safe alternative in selected patients [49]. The patient had no previous abdominal operations and no neglected fasciitis. We recognized the phlegmon and the two complicated diverticula at about 10 cm from each other. An enterectomy was performed with primary anastomosis. The specimen was about 15 cm long, so there was no risk of intestinal failure and small bowel syndrome disease (SBS).

In the second case of accidental detection, we decided on an annual monitoring protocol with clinical examination and CT of the abdomen.

The complexity of our last case was amplified by the dearth of literature available on the subject. While laparoscopic lavage is generally recognized as the gold standard procedure for managing perforated colon diverticulitis, its suitability as a similarly effective and secure option for addressing small bowel diverticula rupture is not yet established. Further research is required to establish the efficacy of laparoscopic lavage in the treatment of these cases. Based on our case and the limited literature on small bowel diverticula, it appears that segmental limited resection with primary anastomosis may be the singular viable option if surgical intervention is necessary.

In both case 2 and case 3, small bowel diverticula were misdiagnosed. These diverticula can be misdiagnosed in radiological examinations due to their small size and the potential for overlap with other structures in the abdomen. One common misdiagnosis of small bowel diverticula is that they are mistaken for small bowel tumors. Due to their similar appearance on imaging studies, such as CT scans and MRIs, small bowel diverticula can be mistakenly identified as tumors, leading to unnecessary biopsies or surgeries. Another potential misdiagnosis is that small bowel diverticula can be overlooked entirely. These tiny pouches may not be easily visible on imaging studies, especially if they are located in obscure areas of the small intestine or if there is poor distention of the bowel during the study. As a result, these diverticula may be missed or dismissed as insignificant findings [48–51]. The accurate diagnosis of small bowel diverticula on radiological examinations can pose a significant challenge to clinicians. As a result, it is imperative for radiologists to remain cognizant of the potential for a misdiagnosis and to meticulously evaluate any small bowel abnormality to ensure that the correct diagnosis is made and appropriate management is administered to the patient. Thus, it is vital for healthcare providers to exercise due diligence and maintain a high level of vigilance when assessing patients with suspected small bowel diverticula [51].

Furthermore, small bowel diverticula can mimic other conditions such as small bowel obstruction or inflammatory bowel disease. This can lead to a delay in the appropriate diagnosis and treatment of the patient.

6. Conclusions

Small bowel diverticula are uncommon but significant medical conditions that require careful monitoring and management. While they may often be asymptomatic, they can lead to serious complications such as bleeding, obstruction, and perforation. Therefore, it is important for surgeons to consider small bowel diverticula as a potential cause of abdominal pain and gastrointestinal symptoms, especially in older patients and in the era of COVID-19.

As we already discussed, the diagnosis of small bowel diverticula can be challenging as they may not always be detected on routine imaging studies. However, advances in imaging technology, such as CT enterography and capsule endoscopy, have improved our ability to identify and characterize these lesions. This, in turn, has led to better understanding of their clinical significance and the potential for intervention.

While surgical intervention has been the traditional treatment approach, further advancement in diagnostic tools may offer less invasive and potentially more effective options. For uncomplicated cases, the management of small bowel diverticula typically involves a combination of dietary modification, symptom control, and surveillance for potential complications.

Strong evidence-based guidelines are needed to guide clinicians in the diagnosis, management, and follow-up of patients with SBNMD. Improving our understanding of this rare condition will lead to better outcomes and quality of life for our patients.

Author Contributions: P.B. was responsible for designing and supervising the study, collecting the data, and writing the manuscript. P.B., N.K., D.K., T.C., A.G. and V.N.P. contributed to writing the manuscript. All authors have read and agreed to the published version of the manuscript.

Funding: This research received no external funding.

Institutional Review Board Statement: The study was conducted according to the Declaration of Helsinki. Ethical review and approval were waived for this study due to the study's retrospective design.

Informed Consent Statement: All patients were required to sign a consent form and be provided with complete information regarding their medical condition, including the proposed treatments, potential risks, and benefits.

Data Availability Statement: The datasets used and analyzed during the current study are available from the corresponding author upon reasonable request.

Conflicts of Interest: The authors declare no conflicts of interest.

Abbreviations

SBNMD	Small bowel non-Meckelian diverticulosis
CT	Computed tomography
SPSS	Statistical package for social science software
SBS	Short bowel syndrome

Appendix A. CARE Checklist

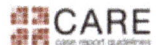

CARE Checklist of information to include when writing a case report

Topic	Item	Checklist item description	Reported on Line
Title	1	The diagnosis or intervention of primary focus followed by the words "case report"	ok
Key Words	2	2 to 5 key words that identify diagnoses or interventions in this case report, including "case report"	ok
Abstract (no references)	3a	Introduction: What is unique about this case and what does it add to the scientific literature?	ok
	3b	Main symptoms and/or important clinical findings	ok
	3c	The main diagnoses, therapeutic interventions, and outcomes	ok
	3d	Conclusion—What is the main "take-away" lesson(s) from this case?	ok
Introduction	4	One or two paragraphs summarizing why this case is unique (may include references)	ok
Patient Information	5a	De-identified patient specific information.	ok
	5b	Primary concerns and symptoms of the patient.	ok
	5c	Medical, family, and psycho-social history including relevant genetic information	ok
	5d	Relevant past interventions with outcomes	ok
Clinical Findings	6	Describe significant physical examination (PE) and important clinical findings.	ok
Timeline	7	Historical and current information from this episode of care organized as a timeline	ok
Diagnostic Assessment	8a	Diagnostic testing (such as PE, laboratory testing, imaging, surveys).	ok
	8b	Diagnostic challenges (such as access to testing, financial, or cultural)	ok
	8c	Diagnosis (including other diagnoses considered)	ok
	8d	Prognosis (such as staging in oncology) where applicable	ok
Therapeutic Intervention	9a	Types of therapeutic intervention (such as pharmacologic, surgical, preventive, self-care)	ok
	9b	Administration of therapeutic intervention (such as dosage, strength, duration)	ok
	9c	Changes in therapeutic intervention (with rationale)	ok
Follow-up and Outcomes	10a	Clinician and patient-assessed outcomes (if available)	ok
	10b	Important follow-up diagnostic and other test results	ok
	10c	Intervention adherence and tolerability (How was this assessed?)	ok
	10d	Adverse and unanticipated events	ok
Discussion	11a	A scientific discussion of the strengths AND limitations associated with this case report	ok
	11b	Discussion of the relevant medical literature with references.	ok
	11c	The scientific rationale for any conclusions (including assessment of possible causes)	ok
	11d	The primary "take-away" lessons of this case report (without references) in a one paragraph conclusion	ok
Patient Perspective	12	The patient should share their perspective in one to two paragraphs on the treatment(s) they received	ok
Informed Consent	13	Did the patient give informed consent? Please provide if requested	Yes ☒ No ☐

References

1. Kassahun, W.T.; Fangmann, J.; Harms, J.; Bartels, M.; Hauss, J. Complicated small-bowel diverticulosis: A case report and review of the literature. *World J. Gastroenterol.* **2007**, *13*, 2240–2242. [CrossRef]
2. Zafouri, E.B.; Ben Ismail, I.; Sghaier, M.; Rebii, S.; Zoghlami, A. Jejunal diverticulitis: A new case report and a review of the literature. *Int. J. Surg. Case Rep.* **2022**, *97*, 73–95. [CrossRef]
3. Harbi, H.; Kardoun, N.; Fendri, S.; Dammak, N.; Toumi, N.; Guirat, A.; Mzali, R. Jejunal diverticulitis. Review and treatment algorithm. *Presse Med.* **2017**, *46*, 1139–1143. [CrossRef]
4. Alam, S.; Rana, A.; Pervez, R. Jejunal diverticulitis: Imaging to management. *Ann. Saudi Med.* **2014**, *34*, 87–90. [CrossRef] [PubMed]
5. Karime, C.; Travers, P.; Ouni, A.; Francis, D. Association between coronavirus disease 2019 and acute Complicated diverticulitis. *Cureus* **2023**, *15*, e33252. [CrossRef] [PubMed]
6. Lebert, P.; Ernst, O.; Zins, M. Acquired diverticular disease of the jejunum and ileum: Imaging features and pitfalls. *Abdom Radiol.* **2019**, *44*, 1734–1743. [CrossRef]
7. Singh, A.K.; Jena, A.; Kumar, P.; Jha, D.K.; Sharma, V. Clinical presentation of COVID 19 in patients with inflammatory bowel disease: A systematic review nad meta-analysis. *Intest Res.* **2022**, *20*, 134–143. [CrossRef] [PubMed]
8. Khsiba, A.; Bradai, S.; Mahmoudi, M.; Mohamed, A.B.; Bradai, J.; Bouzaidi, K.; Mona, M.; Hamzaoui, L.; Azouz, M.M. Jejunal diverticulitis as a rare cause of abdominal pain: A case report. *Pan Afr. Med. J.* **2022**, *41*, 222. [CrossRef]
9. Ben Ismail, I.; Ben Chaabene, H.; Rebii, S.; Zoghlami, A. Perforated Jejunal Diverticulitis: A rare cause of acute abdominal pain. *Clin. Case Rep.* **2021**, *9*, e04594. [CrossRef] [PubMed]
10. Saviano, A.; Brigida, M.; Petruzziello, C.; Zanza, C.; Candelli, M.; Loprete, M.R.M.; Salem, F.; Ojjeti, V. Intestinal damage, inflammation and microbiota alteration during COVID-19 infection. *Biomedicines* **2023**, *11*, 1014. [CrossRef]
11. Delgado-Gonzalez, P.; Gonzalles-Villareal, C.A.; Roacho-Perez, J.A.; Quiros-Reyes, A.G.; Islas, J.F.; Delgado-Gallegos, J.L.; Arellanos-Soto, D.; Galan-Huerta, K.A.; Garza-Trevino, E.N. Inflammatory effect on the gastrointestinal system associated with COVID-19. *World J. Gastroenterol.* **2021**, *27*, 4160–4171. [CrossRef]
12. Aispuro, I.O.; Yazzie, N.P. Diverticulitis of isolated jejunal diverticulum complicated by small bowel obstruction secondary to de novo enterolith formation. *J. Surg. Case Rep.* **2019**, *5*, 151. [CrossRef]
13. Aiyegbeni, B.; Jonnalagadda, S.; Teibe, A. Rare Cause of Left Upper Abdominal Pain. *Prague Med. Rep.* **2021**, *122*, 106–111. [CrossRef]
14. Almalki, M.A.; Yaseen, W.Y.; Baatiyyah, M. Small bowel diverticulum complicated by enterocutaneous fistula and abdominal wall abscess—Case report. *Int. J. Surg. Case Rep.* **2019**, *57*, 39–41. [CrossRef]
15. Anjum, R.; Kumar, N.; Singla, T.; Mani, R.; Karki, B. A Case of Isolated Jejunal Diverticulum Presented as Free Perforation: A Rare Cause of Acute Abdomen. *Cureus* **2021**, *13*, 18809. [CrossRef] [PubMed]
16. Chung, D. Jejunal diverticulosis—A case series and literature review. *Ann. Med. Surg.* **2022**, *75*, 103477. [CrossRef]
17. Coelen, R.J.S.; de Brauw, L.M. Complicated small intestine diverticulitis. *Ned. Tijdschr. Geneeskd.* **2019**, *163*, D3317. [PubMed]
18. De Simone, B.; Alberici, L.; Ansaloni, L.; Sartelli, M.; Coccolini, F.; Catena, F. Not all diverticulitis are colonic: Small bowel diverticulitis—A systematic review. *Minerva Chir.* **2019**, *74*, 137–145. [CrossRef]
19. Di Dier, K.; Van Meerbeeck, S. Ileal Diverticulitis. *J. Belg. Soc. Radiol.* **2023**, *107*, 12. [CrossRef]
20. Duggan, W.P.; Ravi, A.; Chaoudhry, M.A.; Ofori-Kuma, F.; Ivanowski, I. Isolated perforated jejunal diverticulitis: A case report. *J. Surg. Case Rep.* **2021**, *1*, rjaa587. [CrossRef] [PubMed]
21. Elfanagely, Y.; Tse, C.S.; Patil, P.; Lueckel, S. Jejunal Diverticulosis Complicated by Diverticulitis and Small Bowel Obstruction. *Cureus* **2020**, *12*, e8347. [CrossRef] [PubMed]
22. Ghrissi, R.; Harbi, H.; Elghali, M.A.; Belhajkhlifa, M.H.; Letaief, M.R. Jejunal diverticulosis: A rare case of intestinal obstruction. *J. Surg. Case Rep.* **2016**, *2*, rjv176. [CrossRef]
23. Giuffrida, M.; Perrone, G.; Di Saverio, S.; Annicchiarico, A.; Pattonieri, V.; Bonati, E.; Tarasconi, A.; Catena, F. Jejunal diverticulitis: Things to know to prevent diagnostic mistake. *Acta Biomed.* **2021**, *92*, 154.
24. Glaser, J.; Farrel, M.S.; Caplan, R.; Rubino, M. Operative rates in acute diverticulitis with concurrent small bowel obstruction. *Trauma. Surg. Acute Care Open.* **2022**, *7*, e000925. [CrossRef] [PubMed]
25. Hardon, S.F.; den Boer, F.C.; Aallali, T.; Fransen, G.A.; Muller, S. Perforated jejunal diverticula in a young woman: A case report. *Int. J. Surg. Case Rep.* **2021**, *81*, 105838. [CrossRef]
26. Imasato, N.; Kijima, T.; Takada-Owada, A.; Fujita, J.; Takei, K.; Suzuki, I.; Nishihara, D.; Nakamura, T.; Ishida, K.; Kamai, T. Abdominal wall abscess resembling urachal carcinoma caused by ileal diverticulitis. *IJU Case Rep.* **2023**, *6*, 73–76. [CrossRef]
27. Karna, R.; Rana, T.; Mohy-Ud-Din, N.; Chaoudhary, D.; Appasamy, R. Acute hypotensive hematochezia due to jejunal diverticular bleed. *Bayl. Univ. Med Cent. Proc.* **2022**, *35*, 854–855. [CrossRef]
28. Kasuga, Y.; Abe, S.; Nozawa, H.; Sasaki, K.; Murono, K.; Emoto, S.; Matzuzaki, S.; Yokohama, Y.; Nagai, Y.; Yoshioka, Y.; et al. Diverticular perforation of terminal ileum associated with chemotherapy for non-small cell lung carcinoma: A case report. *J. Surg. Case Rep.* **2023**, *2023*, rjad179. [CrossRef]
29. Kunishi, Y.; Kurakami, Y.; Yoshie, K.; Yanagibashi, T.; Oishi, R.; Tsukamoto, M.; Niwa, K.; Kato, Y.; Ota, M.; Maeda, S. Non-surgical management of small bowel diverticulitis with localized perforation: A case report. *Nihon Shokakibyo Gakkai Zasshi.* **2020**, *117*, 327–333.

30. Leigh, N.; Sullivan, B.J.; Anteby, R.; Talbert, S. Perforated jejunal diverticulitis: A rare but important differential in the acute abdomen. *Surg. Case Rep.* **2020**, *6*, 162. [CrossRef] [PubMed]
31. Lutaya, I.; Logvinsky, I.; Mefford, M.; Nway, N.; Qureshi, A. Jejunal-Ileal Diverticulosis Induced Witzel Tube Failure: A Rare Cause of Small Bowel Obstruction. *Cureus* **2022**, *14*, e24209. [CrossRef]
32. Mansour, M.; Abboud, Y.; Bilal, R.; Seilin, N.; Alsuliman, T.; Mohamed, F.K. Small bowel diverticula in elderly patients: A case report and review article. *BMC Surg.* **2022**, *22*, 101. [CrossRef]
33. Matli, V.V.K.; Chandrasekar, V.T.; Campbell, J.L.; Karanam, C.; Jaganmohan, S. Jejunal Diverticulitis: A Rare Diverticular Disease of the Bowel. *Cureus* **2022**, *14*, e21386. [CrossRef]
34. Mendo, R.; Figueiredo, P.; Saldanha, G. Isolated diverticulitis of the terminal ileum: An unusual cause of abdominal pain. *BMJ Case Rep.* **2021**, *14*, e243387. [CrossRef] [PubMed]
35. Cirocchi, R.; Nascimbeni, R.; Burini, G.; Boselli, C.; Barberini, F.; Davies, J.; Di Saverio, S.; Cassini, D.; Amato, B.; Binda, G.A.; et al. The Management of Acute Colonic Diverticulitis in the COVID-19 Era: A Scoping Review. *Medicina* **2021**, *57*, 1127. [CrossRef] [PubMed]
36. Gallo, G.; La Torre, M.; Pietroletti, R.; Bianco, F.; Altomare, D.F.; Pucciarelli, S.; Gagliardi, G.; Perinotti, R. Italian society of colorectal surgery recommendations for good clinical practice in colorectal surgery during the novel coronavirus pandemic. *Tech. Coloproctol.* **2020**, *24*, 501–505. [CrossRef]
37. Uttinger, K.L.; Brunotte, M.; Diers, J.; Lock, J.F.; Jansen-Winkeln, B.; Seehofer, D.; Germer, C.T.; Wiegering, A. Diverticulitis patient care during the COVID-19 pandemic in Germany-a retrospective nationwide population-based cohort study. *Langenbecks Arch. Surg.* **2023**, *408*, 447. [CrossRef]
38. Pajtak, R.; Ramadan, P.; Strauss, P. Strangulated diverticulum: A new acute complication of small bowel diverticulosis. *J. Surg. Case Rep.* **2023**, *2023*, rjad253. [CrossRef] [PubMed]
39. Ponce Beti, M.S.; Palacios Huatako, R.M.; Picco, S.; Capra, A.E.; Perussia, D.G.; Suizer, A.M. Complicated jejunal diverticulosis with intestinal perforation and obstruction: Delay in hospital visit during confinement due to COVID-19. *J. Surg. Case Rep.* **2022**, *2022*, rjac010. [CrossRef]
40. Prough, H.; Jaffe, S.; Jones, B. Jejunal diverticulitis. *J. Surg. Case Rep.* **2019**, *2019*, rjz005. [CrossRef]
41. Rajaguru, K.; Sheong, S.C. Case report on a rare cause of small bowel perforation perforated ileal diverticulum. *Int. J. Surg. Case Rep.* **2021**, *87*, 106465. [CrossRef]
42. Ramzee, A.F.; Khalaf, M.H.; Ahmed, K.; Latif, E.; Aribi, N.; Bouchiba, N.; Singh, R.; Zarour, A. Small Intestinal Diverticulosis: A Rare Cause of Intestinal Perforation Revisited. *Case Rep. Surg.* **2020**, *2020*, 8891521. [CrossRef]
43. Romera-Barba, E.; Galvez Pastor, S.; Navvaro Garcia, M.I.; Torregrosa Perez, N.M.; Sanchez Perez, A.; Vazques Rojas, J.L. Jejunal diverticulosis: A rare cause of intestinal obstruction. *Gastroenterol. Y Hepatol. (Engl. Ed.)* **2017**, *40*, 399–401. [CrossRef]
44. Sammartino, F.; Selvaggio, I.; Montalto, G.M.; Pasesinic, C.; Dhimolea, S.; Krizzuk, D. Acute Abdomen in a 91-Year-Old Male due to Perforated Jejunal Diverticulitis. *Case Rep. Gastroenterol.* **2020**, *14*, 598–603. [CrossRef]
45. Sarıtaş, A.G.; Topal, U.; Eray, C.I.; Dalci, K.; Akcami, A.T.; Erdogan, K. Jejunal diverticulosis complicated with perforation: A rare acute abdomen etiology. *Int. J. Surg. Case Rep.* **2019**, *63*, 101–103. [CrossRef]
46. Vayzband, V.; Ashraf, H.; Esparragoza, P. Surgically Managed Perforated Jejunal Diverticulitis. *Cureus* **2021**, *13*, e15930. [CrossRef]
47. Walter, F.A.; Rimkus, G. Complicated Diverticulitis With Associated Small Bowel Obstruction: A Case Report. *Cureus* **2022**, *14*, e28942. [CrossRef]
48. Watanabe, Y.; Murata, M.; Hirota, M.; Suzuki, R. Whole jejunoileal diverticulosis with recurrent inflammation and perforation: A case report. *Int. J. Surg. Case Rep.* **2021**, *84*, 106020. [CrossRef]
49. Agresta, F.; Ciardo, L.F.; Mazzarolo, G.; Michelet, I.; Orsi, G.; Trentin, G.; Bedin, N. Peritonitis: Laparoscopic approach. *World J. Emerg. Surg.* **2006**, *1*, 9. [CrossRef]
50. Sijberden, J.; Snijders, H.; Van Alteen, S. Laparoscopic lavage in complicated diverticulitis with colonic perforation, Always be closing? *Case Rep. Gastroenterol.* **2021**, *15*, 765–771. [CrossRef]
51. Lamb, R.; Kahion, A.; Sukumar, S.; Layton, B. Small bowel diverticulosis: Imaging apeearences, complications and pitfalls. *Clin. Radiol.* **2022**, *77*, 264–273. [CrossRef] [PubMed]

Disclaimer/Publisher's Note: The statements, opinions and data contained in all publications are solely those of the individual author(s) and contributor(s) and not of MDPI and/or the editor(s). MDPI and/or the editor(s) disclaim responsibility for any injury to people or property resulting from any ideas, methods, instructions or products referred to in the content.

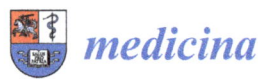

Review

Gastrointestinal Imaging Findings in the Era of COVID-19: A Pictorial Review

Xanthippi Mavropoulou [1,*], Elisavet Psoma [1], Angeliki Papachristodoulou [1,*], Nikoletta Pyrrou [1], Ekaterini Spanou [1], Maria Alexandratou [1], Maria Sidiropoulou [1], Anastasia Theocharidou [1], Vasileios Rafailidis [1], Theofilos Chrysanthidis [2] and Panos Prassopoulos [1]

[1] Department of Clinical Radiology, AHEPA University Hospital of Thessaloniki, Aristotle University of Thessaloniki, 54634 Thessaloniki, Greece; billraf@hotmail.com (V.R.)
[2] Infectious Diseases Division, First Internal Medicine Department, School of Medicine, Aristotle University of Thessaloniki, 54634 Thessaloniki, Greece
* Correspondence: xmavropoulou@gmail.com (X.M.); angeliquep321@gmail.com (A.P.)

Abstract: The potentially fatal COVID-19 pandemic has been associated with a largespectrum of clinical presentations. Beyond the classical pulmonary manifestations, gastrointestinal tract-related symptoms suchas nausea, diarrhea, abdominal distention and pain have been observed in patients, as a consequence of the binding of SARS-CoV-19 to Angiotensin-converting Enzyme 2 (ACE2) receptors in the gastrointestinal (GI) tract. The early recognition ofspecific imaging features, including hepatobiliary involvement, pancreatic involvement, development of solid organ infarcts, ischemic bowel changes and vascular occlusion, plays a key role through the course of the disease. Also, suspicious symptoms, especially in critically ill patients with clinical and biochemical markers of hypovolemia, necessitate timely imaging for bleeding complications. The aim of this pictorial review is to illustrate the spectrum of the GIimaging findings in patients with COVID-19. Awareness of diagnostic imaging hallmarks is crucial to optimize the management of these patients.

Keywords: COVID-19; abdominal; gastrointestinal; CT/CTA; pancreatitis; colitis cholecystitis; pancreatitis; bleeding

Citation: Mavropoulou, X.; Psoma, E.; Papachristodoulou, A.; Pyrrou, N.; Spanou, E.; Alexandratou, M.; Sidiropoulou, M.; Theocharidou, A.; Rafailidis, V.; Chrysanthidis, T.; et al. Gastrointestinal Imaging Findings in the Era of COVID-19: A Pictorial Review. *Medicina* **2023**, *59*, 1332. https://doi.org/10.3390/medicina59071332

Academic Editors: Ludovico Abenavoli and Giovanni Tarantino

Received: 15 May 2023
Revised: 3 July 2023
Accepted: 4 July 2023
Published: 19 July 2023

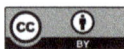

Copyright: © 2023 by the authors. Licensee MDPI, Basel, Switzerland. This article is an open access article distributed under the terms and conditions of the Creative Commons Attribution (CC BY) license (https://creativecommons.org/licenses/by/4.0/).

1. Introduction

Since December 2019, the world has observed the appearance and spread of SARS-CoV-19, a novel coronavirus that causes a severe respiratory syndrome (COVID-19) and its disastrous impact on global health [1,2]. COVID-19 was declared as a pandemic on March 11, 2020 by the World Health Organization (WHO), and since then millions of people worldwide have been affected. As of May 2023, more than six million deaths have been confirmed.

Although in the majority of cases, the disease manifests with respiratory symptoms such as cough, fever and dyspnea, its extra-pulmonary manifestations are being increasingly acknowledged [3] Specifically, the incidence of GI manifestations such as abdominal pain, nausea or diarrhea has ranged from 12% to as much as 61% in patients with COVID-19. Moreover, some patients might present only with GI symptoms, hindering diagnosis. Furthermore, it has been noted that patients presenting with GI symptoms tend to progress more to a severe form of disease with poor outcomes [4–6]. As it is well documented that SARS-CoV-19 uses ACE-2 receptors to enter human cells, this receptor is found to be expressed not only in pulmonary epithelial cells but also in gastrointestinal and hepatobiliary cells, explaining the GI involvement [7,8]. Despite the broad recognition of respiratory imaging findings, until now few studies have been published about abdominal radiological presentation of patients with COVID-19 [9,10].

Taking into consideration the high possibility of GI tract involvement, it is crucial for radiologists to be aware of the variety of abdominal imaging findings in patients with COVID-19, as early recognition can aid the diagnosis in patients with nonspecific, atypical symptoms.

2. Materials and Methods

The aim of this study is to share our experience and present the imaging findings of GI manifestations that can be noted in patients with COVID 19.

The authors executed a retrospective study from our hospital archives starting from February 2020, when the first COVID-19 patient was admitted in our hospital, until 31 December of 2022. Six of the authors searched the institutional databases of COVID-19 patients who underwent abdominal CT. Confirmed COVID-19 patients who presented with abdominal signs and symptoms were included in the study. A dedicated 16-slice SIEMENS EMOTION CT scanner was used for confirmed COVID-19 cases. The final study population was 84 patients. Simultaneously, a search of the published literature was conducted on PubMed using suitable key words (e.g., COVID-19, abdominal manifestations, CT, imaging, and gastrointestinal).

2.1. Colon Manifestations

The bowel is the most commonly involved abdominal organ in COVID-19 patients. Frequent abdominal imaging features include intestinal imaging findings (24%), including colorectal (5%) and small bowel thickening (12%), intestinal distension (18%), pneumatosis and intestinal perforation [11]. Bhayana R. et al. observed [9] similar bowel-wall abnormalities in 31% of CT images in patients in the Intensive Care Unit (ICU). Common indications for CT evaluation include abdominal pain or distention, hematochezia and nausea [3]. It is important to note that the presence of bowel abnormalities predict worse prognosis and increased clinical severity.

ACE 2 receptors are located in gastrointestinal cells (enterocytes and vascular cells) and can interpret the bowel manifestations of the virus, specifically the inflammatory bowel manifestations and ischemic bowel alterations. This is supported by the detection of SARS-CoV-19 virus in feces samples [4,12]. Infection of the GI tract epithelial cells is followed by an inflammatory response and a cytokine release.

A large bowel infection usually appears with diffuse circumferential and enhancing wall thickening (hyperenhancement) that can involve one or more segments of the colon (Figures 1 and 2). Pericolic fluid or perintestinal fat stranding is common while pericolic lymphadenopathy is not (Figures 3 and 4). If we suspect COVID-19-related colitis, clinical correlation is needed, and the detection of the virus in stools can establish the diagnosis.

It is very important to suspect and diagnose patients presenting acute mesenteric ischemia (AMI) or perforation of the bowel [13]. It is well documented that critically ill COVID-19 patients are at risk for thrombosis or bleeding [14].

AMI, is associated with severe symptoms, a worsening systemic status and high morbidity and mortality. Imaging has a crucial role in its detection and is the cornerstone of diagnosis [15]. An ultrasound is nonspecific with low sensitivity but may reveal decreased peristalsis and intraluminal content that indicate stasis.

CT angiography remains the pillar for detection of signs of ischemia [16]. Filling defects that represent emboli or thrombi within the lumen of the abdominal aorta and its branches are major findings along with hypoenhancement of the mesenteric vascular arcade and decreased contrast enhancement of the bowel wall that indicates hypoperfusion. In some cases, a target appearance of the bowel wall, representing mucosal hyperemia with adjacent mural edema, can be depicted in ischemic colitis. The affected segment appears with thickened bowel walls, and it may be pictured as fluid-filled due to disruption of peristalsis [17]. Additional findings are porto-mesenteric venous gas, pneumatosis intestinalis and pneumoperitoneum [18,19]. In a later phase, the bowel wall is thinned due to loss of normal tone.

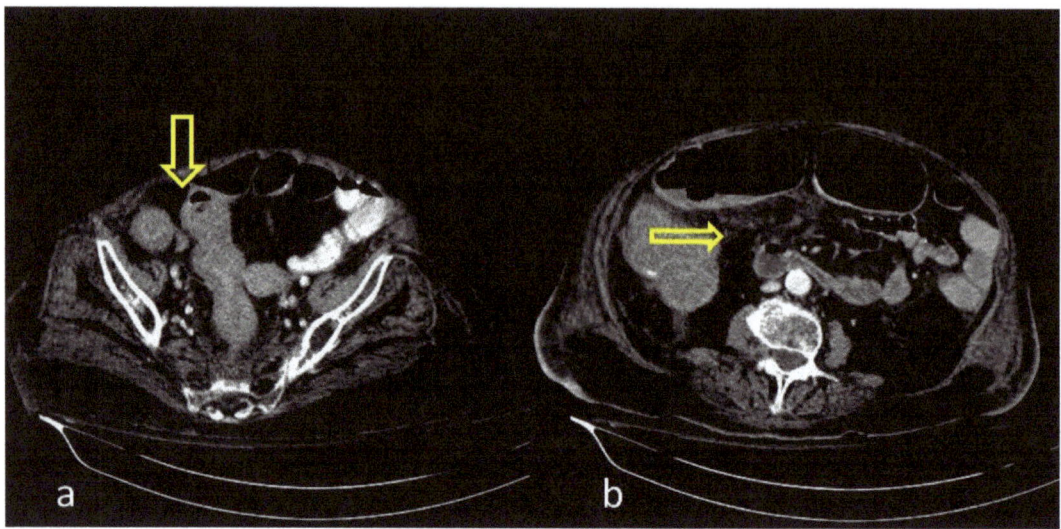

Figure 1. COVID-19 (+) hospitalized 75-year-old male patient with abdominal pain and diarrhea. Abdominal Contrast Enhanced CT (CECT) depicted bowel wall thickening ((**a**), thick arrow) and mesenteric fat stranding ((**b**), thin arrow). The imaging findings are indicative of inflammatory colitis.

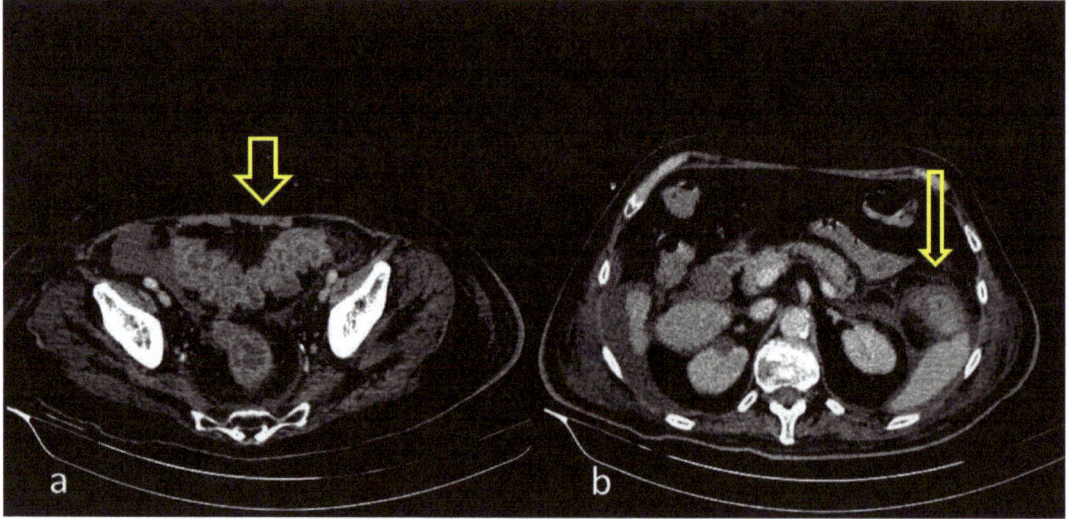

Figure 2. COVID-19 (+) 68-year-old patient with a long hospital stay was subjected to an abdominal CECT for acute abdominal pain, which showed colonic wall thickening ((**a**), thick arrow) and adjacent fat stranding ((**b**), thin arrow).

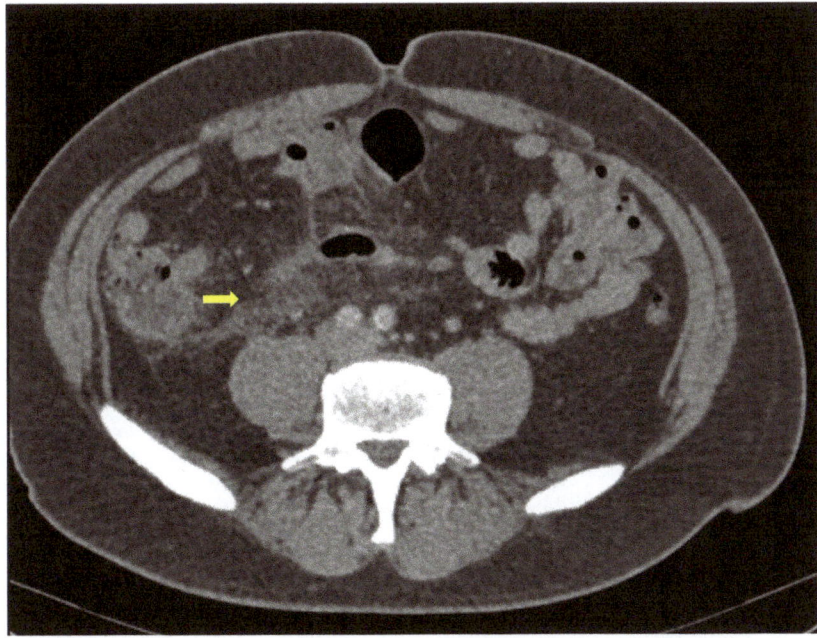

Figure 3. 55-year-old male patient with COVID-19 pneumonia with right lower quadrant pain. CT on admission demonstrating a thickened appendix and proximal fat stranding (yellow arrow), indicating acute appendicitis.

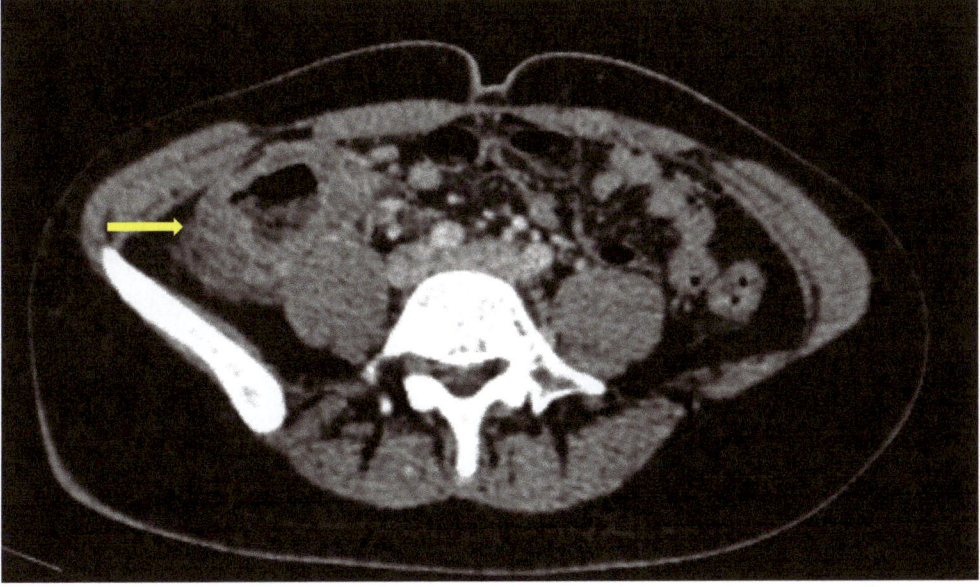

Figure 4. A 48-year-old female patient with COVID-19 pneumonia and no other comorbidities. CT scan depicted a thickened cecum with proximal fat stranding (yellow arrow).

2.2. Small Intestine Manifestations

When COVID-19 affects the small intestine, it can cause a range of symptoms, including diarrhea, abdominal pain and vomiting, in both adults and children [20].

One study published in the Journal of Medical Virology examined the fecal samples of COVID-19 patients and found that the virus was present in the samples of 23 out of 29 patients, indicating that SARS-CoV-19 can be transmitted via the fecal–oral route. Additionally, the virus was present in higher amounts in patients with gastrointestinal symptoms, such as diarrhea and nausea [21].

Another study found that nearly half of COVID-19 patients had gastrointestinal symptoms, such as diarrhea, nausea and vomiting. Those patients experienced a longer duration of illness compared to those without digestive symptoms [22].

The exact mechanisms by which COVID-19 affects the small intestine are still not fully understood, but it is thought that the virus may directly infect the intestinal cells or that it may cause an inflammatory response that affects the gut. Additionally, some patients may experience a dysregulated immune response, which can also contribute to small bowel manifestations, including inflammation, mucosal injury and microthrombi formation [23].

Several studies have investigated the CT findings associated with small intestine involvement. In the CT scans of 149 COVID-19 patients, nearly 20% were indicative of small intestine involvement, with wall thickening, luminal dilatation and mucosal enhancement, especially in severe cases associated with worse outcomes (Figure 5) [22].

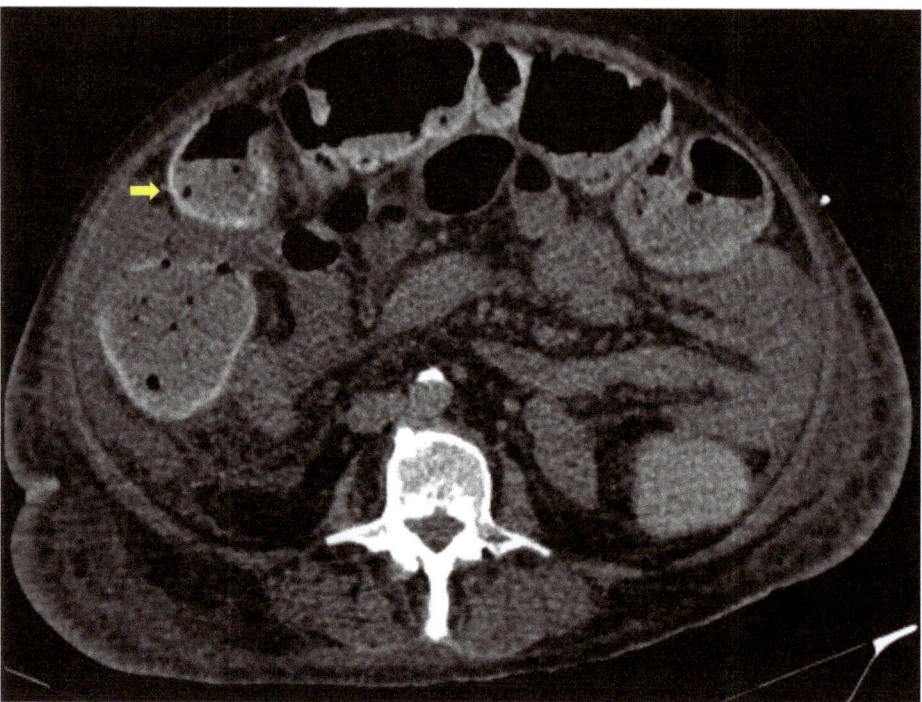

Figure 5. 59-year-old female patient with severe COVID-19 pneumonia hospitalized in the ICU. CT demonstrating distended large bowel with hyperenhanced walls and free abdominal fluid (shock bowel)—yellow arrow. Note the concomitant subcutaneous edema.

Bhayana et al. found that 29% of CTs showed bowel wall thickening involving the colon or small bowel, such as findings of ischemia with pneumatosis or portal venous gas and bowel perforation and a fluid-filled colon in 43% of patients, suggestive of diarrhea.

In addition to small bowel abnormalities, (Figure 6) CT imaging has also shown evidence of mesenteric lymphadenopathy, with mesenteric lymph node enlargement and increased enhancement in 22% of patients [9].

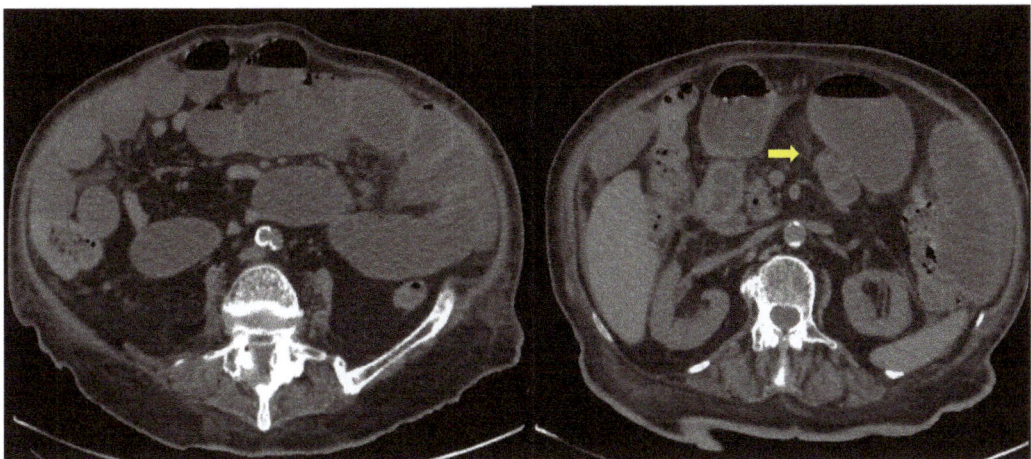

Figure 6. 85-year old-patient with small bowel ileus (fluid filled loops—yellow arrow) at the 4th day of hospitalization.

However, as these findings are not specific, CT findings must be correlated with clinical and laboratory data to confirm a COVID-19 diagnosis.

2.3. Hepato-Biliary Involvement

ACE2 receptors are found in many organs including the liver and biliary system, thus giving the opportunity for a local inflammation of these organs [24].

The hepatobiliary involvement in patients with COVID-19 infection and the abdominal imaging findings in those patients represent an interesting topic for further investigation.

One of the most common imaging findings in CT examinations of COVID-19 patients with hepatobiliary dysfunction (both in the literature and in our series) is hepatomegaly with or without a diffuse decrease in liver/spleen attenuation ratio. This can be due to liver injury due to the virus, pre-existing comorbidities (obesity, nonalcoholic fatty liver, and hepatitis) or as a result of hospitalization (parenteral nutrition and hepatotoxic drugs) [25,26].

In severe cases of COVID-19 infection, mostly in patients in ICU, a heterogenicity and mosaic pattern of the liver parenchyma is seen, combined with periportal edema and a contrast reflux in dilated hepatic veins indicating liver congestion due to hypoxia and cardiac failure [25].

Biliary imaging findings are also encountered in patients with COVID-19 infection. In our institution, many patients presented with right quadrant pain and nausea/vomiting after a meal. In ultrasound and CT examinations, the findings included gallbladder distention, wall thickening and mural edema, pericholecystic fluid and inflammatory fat stranding with calculi and/or sludge (Figures 7 and 8).

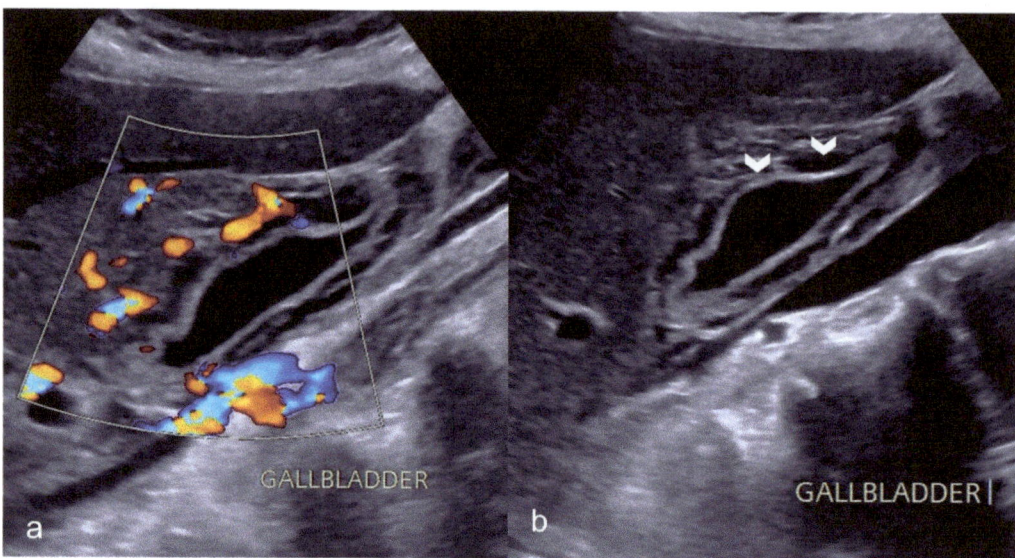

Figure 7. A 69-year-old man with COVID-19 presented a positive Murphy sign. Ultrasound images showed gallbladder wall striation and increased thickness ((**b**)-arrowheads). The Color Doppler technique revealed hyperemia (**a**). No gallbladder stones were present indicating acalculous cholecystitis.

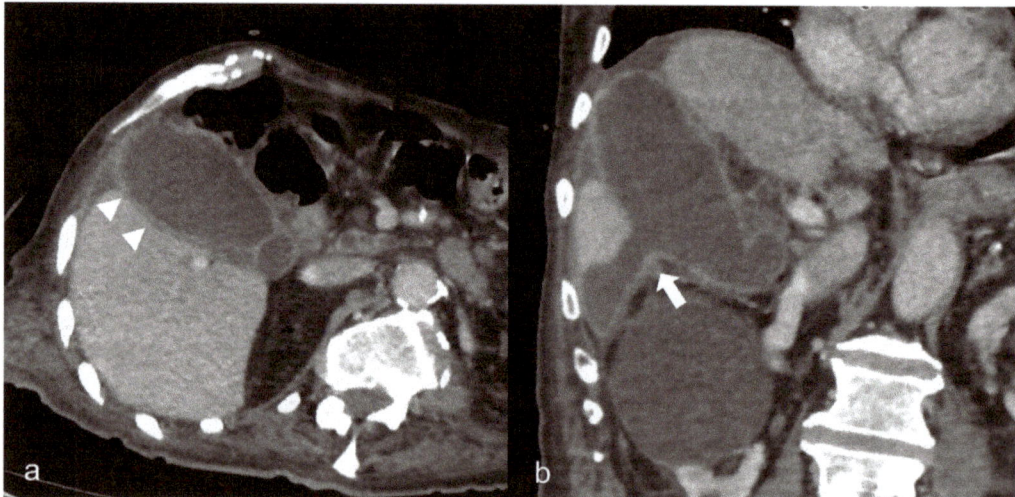

Figure 8. A 90-year-old COVID-19 patient presented acute right quadrant abdominal pain and cholestasis. Computed tomography on the axial (**a**) and coronal (**b**) plane showed acute cholecystitis with diffuse thickening of the gallbladder wall and pericholecystic fluid (arrowheads). Disruption of the gallbladder wall (arrow) is also present with fluid collection around the liver indicating perforation.

Less frequently, acalculous cholecystitis with sludge is seen in patients in the ICU, indicating cholestasis due to parenteral nutrition and/ or systemic inflammation [27,28].

2.4. Pancreatic Involvement

The data on pancreatic involvement during SARS-CoV-19 infection are limited. The frequency and severity of pancreatic damage and acute pancreatitis (AP) and its pathophysiology are still being studied.

AP is usually caused by increased alcohol consumption and gallstones. However, in 10%–20% of cases, an etiological factor cannot be identified [29]. A number of infectious agents, such as Coxsackie B virus and hepatitis A virus, infect the pancreas [30]. Radiology and imaging findings play a vital role mainly in the detection and follow up of complications of AP [30].

According to the revised Atlanta classification, the diagnosis of AP requires two of the following: (a) typical abdominal pain, (b) a serum lipase level (or amylase) at least three times greater than the upper normal limit and (c) characteristic imaging findings on CT, MRI or ultrasonography [31].

A study performed in pigeons with severe pancreatitis has managed to isolate COVID-19 or a Coronavirus-like virus, but no similar studies have been conducted in humans [32]. SARS-COV-19 uses ACE-2 receptors to enter pancreatic ductal cells [33], a fact that could explain the infection of the gland. Another possible way to induce the pancreatic injury is the caused cytokine storm, which produces pancreatic inflammation and an uncontrolled inflammatory immune systemic response caused by COVID-19. Finally, another important cause is the drug-induced pancreatic injury from antivirals, non-steroidal anti-inflammatory drugs (NSAIDs), tocilizumab and baricitinib, which belong to the approved treatment of COVID-19 [4].

Amylase and lipase elevation has been reported in 8.5–17.3% of patients with COVID-19. However, those enzymes are also increased in other gastrointestinal diseases, such as gastritis and colitis that have also been reported in COVID-19 patients. A meta-analysis of patients with COVID-19 showed that 18% had gastrointestinal symptoms and raised pancreatic enzymes could not be directly associated with pancreatitis [34]. Furthermore, kidneys play a major role in the clearance of both amylase and lipase, and their insufficiency could result in the elevation of these enzymes [35]. It has been proved that COVID-19 can infect insulin-producing cells in the pancreas and change their function, potentially explaining the high privilege of diabetes in previously healthy individuals [36].

The temporal relationship between the onset of COVID-19 infection and inflammation of the pancreas has not been clearly established. Some patients develop COVID-19 symptoms and abdominal pain when the infection begins, whereas others present with AP several days after COVID-19 diagnosis (Figure 9) [37].

A study of 52 patients with COVID-19 pneumonia showed that there was a 17% incidence of pancreatic injury. Kumar V. et al. studied patients with acute pancreatitis and COVID-19 infection and found that half of them developed AP after a median of 22.5 days from the onset of respiratory symptoms, while the rest of them were admitted for abdominal pain [38] Another systematic review, including overall 37 patients, summarized that AP might be the first symptom of COVID-19 [39]. In addition, COVID-19 may negatively influence the morbidity and mortality linked with AP [40].

Finally, it should be noted that after the COVID-19 pandemic, pancreatic cancer and metastases rates have been dramatically raised, as there was a temporary cessation of screening during the pandemic. Less than 25% of patients had regular availability of diagnostic and staging tools, while 20% were unable to perform surgery [41].

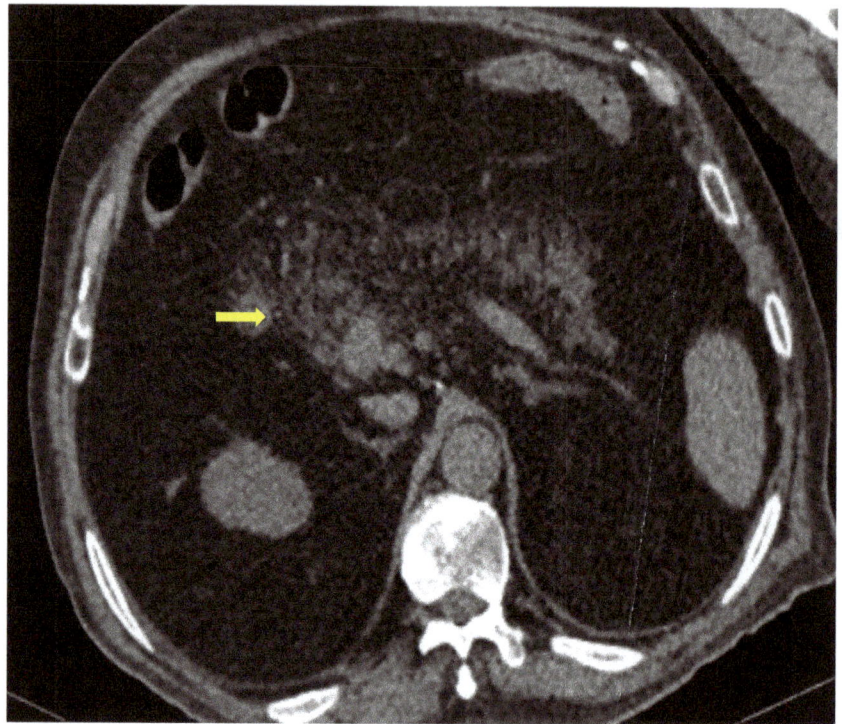

Figure 9. 81-year-old patient with COVID-19 pneumonia developed epigastric pain at the second day of hospitalization. CT demonstrating acute pancreatitis (yellow arrow).

2.5. Thromboembolic Complications

Systemic coagulopathy is common in COVID-19 patients with severe pneumonia [42].

Despite the limited available data, many thrombotic manifestations regarding the abdominal vessels have been documented in cases of COVID-19 inpatients. The CT depiction frequency is highly dependent on the performed protocol, which is usually unenhanced or contains only a portal venous phase. Only in a few cases the image acquisition is accomplished through an abdominal multiphase CT angiogram. Consequently, thromboembolic events regarding the arterial abdominal branches are scarcely reported, opposed to venous thrombi, possibly due to underdiagnosis [43].

In many cases we can only depict indirect findings due to the small vessel thrombotic nature of the disease, a phenomenon that could also be related to hospitalization or comorbidities [11]. When it comes to microvasculature, both arteries and veins are affected [44]. An interesting fact is that in an accountable percentage of the arterial thrombi, the affected vessels did not have any atherosclerotic alterations, suggesting that COVID-19 was the generating factor of the thrombus [45].

Solid abdominal organs infarcts have been documented during imaging protocols performed for pulmonary embolism detection, especially in patients with elevation of the D-dimers. Apart from those cases, renal infarcts were reported in scans performed for vague abdominal pain or due to acute kidney failure [45].

Fewer reports about splenic infracts in COVID-19 patients also come from thoracic scans with abdominal extension [46].

A single-center small retrospective study reported in COVID-19 patients 15 cases of acute aortic thrombosis, splenic artery thrombosis (associated with splenic infraction), superior mesenteric and renal artery thrombosis such as a celiac and an internal iliac thrombosis. An interesting part was a patient with infrarenal aortic wall inflammation and focal dissection, while many venous thromboses have been described (affecting the portal vein, inferior, superior mesenteric, renal, ovarian vein and inferior vena cava). Reports of indirect findings of the splanchnic branch venous occlusion described bowel wall severe edema, hyperenhancement or severe hypoenhancement, associated mesenteric and portal intravenous gas, bowel pneumatosis and pneumoperitoneum (Figure 10) [47]. Bari Dane et al. published a case of a simultaneous nonocclusive aortic, celiac and superior mesenteric artery thrombus combined with a complete common hepatic artery thrombus [48].

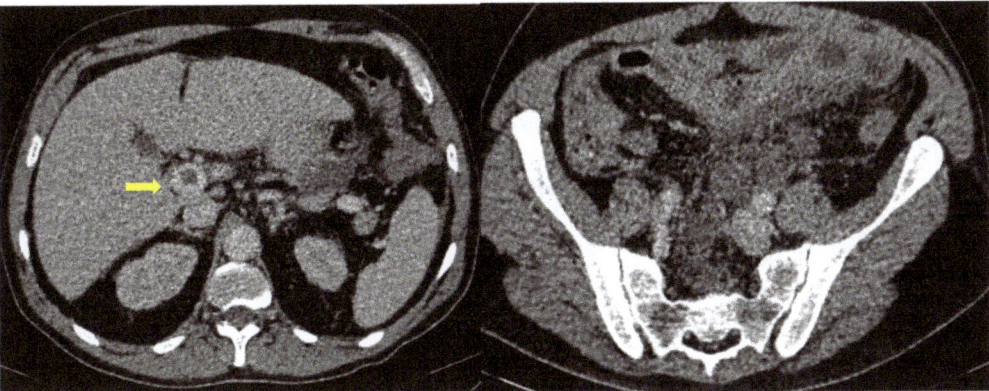

Figure 10. 56-year-old hospitalized male patient with COVID-19 pneumonia with raised level of d-dimers. CT depicting the thrombosed portal vein (yellow arrow). Note that in the same scan, there is extended small bowel thickening with mesenteric free fluid.

Those findings are in accordance with reports of bowel pneumatosis as a thrombotic event outcome [49], while many case reports and large case series demonstrate major abdominal—both arterial and venous—thrombosis in COVID-19 patients. In fact, many patients suffer from thrombotic occlusion despite prophylaxis or even the full-dose anticoagulation therapy supporting evidence of COVID-19 direct endothelial injury [50].

2.6. Bleeding Manifestations

Bleeding in patients with COVID-19 can be the result of pre-existing risks factors, antithrombotic drugs and a massive immune response to the virus, [51]. A common bleeding complication is abdominal hematomas, usually of the Iliopsoas and rectus abdominis muscle [51,52]. The role of a CT scan is major in both the diagnosis and treatment of these entities. They are usually seen as muscle enlargement with increased densities, blood-fluid level and possibly extravasation of contrast. When it comes to the GI tract, upper GI is the most common site of bleeding followed by the lower GI [53,54].

A potential pathogenic route is through the binding of the virus with Angiotensin Converting Enzyme-2 expressed in gastrointestinal epithelial cells [55].

Underlying mucosal lesions in the GI (ulcers and vascular abnormalities) and prophylactic/therapeutic anticoagulant therapy should be considered and further investigated.

GI hemorrhage is less commonly encountered in abdominal imaging, and CT findings include active intraluminal extravasation of contrast and indirect signs such as luminal distention with blood clots (Figure 11) [56].

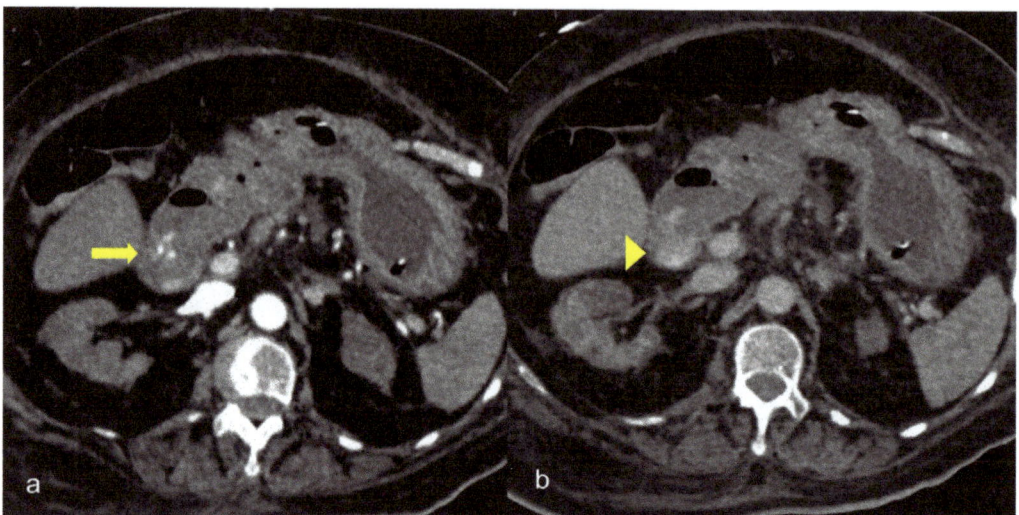

Figure 11. A 75-year-old intubated patient with COVID-19 presented with hematemesis, hypotension and acute drop of hemoglobin level. Computed Tomography revealed active intraluminal extravasation of contrast into the 2nd part of duodenum (arrow) on arterial phase (**a**). Further pooling of the contrast (arrowhead) is shown on portal phase (**b**).

Imaging is additionally significant to the treatment plan by identifying the exact site and extent of the bleeding as well as offering a precise and minimally invasive treatment option. Digital Subtraction Angiography can confirm the active bleeding seen as a "contrast blush", detect the responsible branch and provide occlusion via selective embolization.

3. Results

In our institution, 84 COVID-19 patients underwent abdominal CT imaging studies displaying positive GI imaging findings. The study population included 43 males and 41 females. The oldest patient was 90 years old, and the youngest patient was 18 years old. Fourteen patients were admitted to the ICU, and in total 26 patients died.

The most frequent indications for abdominal CT were abdominal pain and abdominal distention. The majority of the patients presented elevated levels of liver enzymes and C reactive protein.

The most frequent comorbidities included hypertension, heart disease, dyslipidemia, diabetes mellitus, obesity and cancer. Also, a patient with kidney transplant was included.

The most common imaging findings concerned the small intestine and colon. Bowel wall thickening was noted in 25 patients (22 of them in colorectal area and the rest in small bowel) accompanied with pericolic fluid (6 patients), submucosal edema (6 patients) or intestinal perforation (2 patients). Furthermore, thrombosis of SMA was noted in one patient.

Hepatobiliary manifestations were also common with 22 patients presenting liver steatosis, 3 patients suffering from acute cholecystitis and 24 patients in total presenting biliary sludge and/or gallstones.

Seven patients experienced pancreatitis during their hospitalization.

In our institution, we are in concordance with the few publications about the abdominal manifestations of COVID-19. It was not our intention to present a statistical analysis of our findings but to expound upon the plethora of imaging findings in regard to the digestive system involvement.

In the future, a more extensive study and analysis should take place, in collaboration with other tertiary referral centers, using a bigger sample.

4. Conclusions

COVID-19 is a multi-organ disease, and GI manifestation might be noted at the time of diagnosis or later in the course of the disease. The presence of GI manifestations is associated with increased clinical severity and poor outcome. Therefore, it is pivotal for radiologists to be aware of related imaging findings to aid diagnosis and appropriate management.

Author Contributions: Conceptualization: X.M., E.P. and V.R. Methodology: X.M., A.P., N.P., E.S., M.A., M.S. and A.T. Software, data curation, formal analysis, investigation, writing—original draft preparation: A.P., N.P., E.S., M.A., M.S. and A.T. Validation: X.M. Resources: T.C. Supervision: P.P. Project administration X.M. All authors have read and agreed to the published version of the manuscript.

Funding: This research received no external funding.

Institutional Review Board Statement: Ethical review and approval were waived for this study due to the retrospective nature of the study including non-identifying images acquired for clinically indicated reasons.

Informed Consent Statement: Informed consent acquired by all patients presented.

Data Availability Statement: Not available due to confidentiality of imaging examinations.

Conflicts of Interest: The authors declare no conflict of interest.

References

1. Wang, H.; Wei, R.; Rao, G.; Zhu, J.; Song, B. Characteristic CT Findings Distinguishing 2019 Novel Coronavirus Disease (COVID-19) from Influenza Pneumonia. *Eur. Radiol.* **2020**, *30*, 4910–4917. [CrossRef] [PubMed]
2. Yang, W.; Cao, Q.; Qin, L.; Wang, X.; Cheng, Z.; Pan, A.; Dai, J.; Sun, Q.; Zhao, F.; Qu, J.; et al. Clinical characteristics and imaging manifestations of the 2019 novel coronavirus disease (COVID-19):A multi-center study in Wenzhou city, Zhejiang, China. *J. Infect.* **2020**, *80*, 388–393. [CrossRef] [PubMed]
3. Gupta, A.; Madhavan, M.V.; Sehgal, K.; Nair, N.; Mahajan, S.; Sehrawat, T.S.; Bikdeli, B.; Ahluwalia, N.; Ausiello, J.C.; Wan, E.Y.; et al. Extrapulmonary manifestations of COVID-19. *Nat. Med.* **2020**, *26*, 1017–1032. [CrossRef]
4. Tian, Y.; Rong, L.; Nian, W.; He, Y. Review article: Gastrointestinal features in COVID-19 and the possibility of faecal transmission. *Aliment. Pharmacol. Ther.* **2020**, *51*, 843–851. [CrossRef]
5. Redd, W.D.; Zhou, J.C.; Hathorn, K.E.; McCarty, T.R.; Bazarbashi, A.N.; Thompson, C.C.; Shen, L.; Chan, W.W. Prevalence and Characteristics of Gastrointestinal Symptoms in Patients With Severe Acute Respiratory Syndrome Coronavirus 2 Infection in the United States: A Multicenter Cohort Study. *Gastroenterology* **2020**, *159*, 765–767.e2. [CrossRef] [PubMed]
6. Mao, R.; Qiu, Y.; He, J.S.; Tan, J.Y.; Li, X.H.; Liang, J.; Shen, J.; Zhu, L.-R.; Chen, Y.; Iacucci, M.; et al. Manifestations and prognosis of gastrointestinal and liver involvement in patients with COVID-19: A systematic review and meta-analysis. *Lancet Gastroenterol. Hepatol.* **2020**, *5*, 667–678. [CrossRef]
7. Li, G.; He, X.; Zhang, L.; Ran, Q.; Wang, J.; Xiong, A.; Wu, D.; Chen, F.; Sun, J.; Chang, C. Assessing ACE2 expression patterns in lung tissues in the pathogenesis of COVID-19. *J. Autoimmun.* **2020**, *112*, 102463. [CrossRef]
8. Hamming, I.; Timens, W.; Bulthuis, M.L.C.; Lely, A.T.; Navis, G.J.; van Goor, H. Tissue distribution of ACE2 protein, the functional receptor for SARS coronavirus. A first step in understanding SARS pathogenesis. *J. Pathol.* **2004**, *203*, 631–637. [CrossRef]
9. Bhayana, R.; Som, A.; Li, M.D.; Carey, D.E.; Anderson, M.A.; Blake, M.A.; Catalano, O.; Gee, M.S.; Hahn, P.F.; Harisinghani, M.; et al. Abdominal imaging findings in COVID-19: Preliminary observations. *Radiology* **2020**, *297*, E207–E215. [CrossRef]
10. Guo, Y.; Hu, X.; Yu, F.; Chen, J.; Zheng, W.; Liu, J.; Zeng, P. Abdomen CT findings in a COVID-19 patient with intestinal symptoms and possibly false negative RT-PCR before initial discharge. *Quant. Imaging Med. Surg.* **2020**, *10*, 1158–1161. [CrossRef]
11. Horvat, N.; Pinto, P.V.; Araujo-Filho, J.D.; Santos, J.M.; Dias, A.B.; Miranda, J.A.; de Oliveira, C.V.; Barbosa, C.S.; Morais, T.C.; Assuncao, A.N., Jr.; et al. Abdominal gastrointestinal imaging findings on computed tomography in patients with COVID-19 and correlation with clinical outcomes. *Eur. J. Radiol. Open* **2021**, *8*, 100326. [CrossRef] [PubMed]
12. Xiao, F.; Tang, M.; Zheng, X.; Liu, Y.; Li, X.; Shan, H. Evidence for Gastrointestinal Infection of SARS-CoV-2. *Gastroenterology* **2020**, *158*, 1831–1833.e3. [CrossRef] [PubMed]
13. Childers, B.C.; Cater, S.W.; Horton, K.M.; Fishman, E.K.; Johnson, P.T. CT evaluation of acute enteritis and colitis: Is it infectious, inflammatory, or ischemic? *Radiographics* **2015**, *35*, 1940–1941. [CrossRef] [PubMed]
14. Tang, N.; Li, D.; Wang, X.; Sun, Z. Abnormal coagulation parameters are associated with poor prognosis in patients with novel coronavirus pneumonia. *J. Thromb. Haemost.* **2020**, *18*, 844–847. [CrossRef] [PubMed]
15. Parry, A.H.; Wani, A.H.; Yaseen, M. Acute Mesenteric Ischemia in Severe Coronavirus-19 (COVID-19): Possible Mechanisms and Diagnostic Pathway. *Acad. Radiol.* **2020**, *27*, 1190. [CrossRef]

16. Furukawa, A.; Kanasaki, S.; Kono, N.; Wakamiya, M.; Tanaka, T.; Takahashi, M.; Murata, K. CT diagnosis of acute mesenteric ischemia from various causes. *Am. J. Roentgenol.* **2009**, *192*, 408–416. [CrossRef]
17. Taourel, P.G.; Deneuville, M.; Pradel, J.; Régent, D.; Bruel, J.M. Acute Mesenteric Ischemia: Diagnosis with Contrast-enhanced CT'. *Radiology* **1996**, *199*, 632–636. [CrossRef]
18. Corrêa Neto, I.J.F.; Viana, K.F.; Silva, M.B.S.d.; Silva, L.M.d.; Oliveira, G.d.; Cecchini, A.R.d.; Rolim, A.S.; Robles, L. Perforated acute abdomen in a patient with COVID-19: An atypical manifestation of the disease. *J. Coloproctol.* **2020**, *40*, 269–272. [CrossRef]
19. De Nardi, P.; Parolini, D.C.; Ripa, M.; Racca, S.; Rosati, R. Bowel perforation in a Covid-19 patient: Case report. *Int. J. Color. Dis.* **2020**, *35*, 1797–1800. [CrossRef]
20. Behzad, S.; Aghaghazvini, L.; Radmard, A.R.; Gholamrezanezhad, A. Extrapulmonary manifestations of COVID-19: Radiologic and clinical overview. *Clin. Imaging* **2020**, *66*, 35–41. [CrossRef]
21. Chen, Y.; Chen, L.; Deng, Q.; Zhang, G.; Wu, K.; Ni, L.; Yang, Y.; Liu, B.; Wang, W.; Wei, C.; et al. The presence of SARS-CoV-2 RNA in the feces of COVID-19 patients. *J. Med. Virol.* **2020**, *92*, 833–840. [CrossRef] [PubMed]
22. Pan, L.; Mu, M.; Yang, P.; Sun, Y.; Wang, R.; Yan, J.; Li, P.; Hu, B.; Wang, J.; Hu, C.; et al. Clinical characteristics of COVID-19 patients with digestive symptoms in Hubei, China: A descriptive, cross-sectional, multicenter study. *Am. J. Gastroenterol.* **2020**, *115*, 766–773. [CrossRef] [PubMed]
23. Zhang, H.; Kang, Z.; Gong, H.; Xu, D.; Wang, J.; Li, Z.; Cui, X.; Xiao, J.; Meng, T.; Zhou, W.; et al. The digestive system is a potential route of 2019-nCov infection: A bioinformatics 1 analysis based on single-cell transcriptomes 2. *bioRxiv* **2020**. [CrossRef]
24. Abdelmohsen, M.A.; Alkandari, B.M.; Gupta, V.K.; ElBeheiry, A.A. Diagnostic value of abdominal sonography in confirmed COVID-19 intensive care patients. *Egypt. J. Radiol. Nucl. Med.* **2020**, *51*, 198. [CrossRef]
25. Sodeifian, F.; Seyedalhosseini, Z.S.; Kian, N.; Eftekhari, M.; Najari, S.; Mirsaeidi, M.; Farsi, Y.; Nasiri, M.J. Drug-Induced Liver Injury in COVID-19 Patients: A Systematic Review. Frontiers in Medicine. *Front. Media* **2021**, *8*, 731436. [CrossRef]
26. Metawea, M.I.; Yousif, W.I.; Moheb, I. COVID 19 and liver: An A–Z literature review. *Dig. Liver Dis.* **2021**, *53*, 146–152. [CrossRef]
27. Mattone, E.; Sofia, M.; Schembari, E.; Palumbo, V.; Bonaccorso, R.; Randazzo, V.; La Greca, G.; Iacobello, C.; Russello, D.; Latteri, S. Acute acalculous cholecystitis on a COVID-19 patient: A case report. *Ann. Med. Surg.* **2020**, *58*, 73–75. [CrossRef]
28. Mossaab, G.; Ben Khlifa, M.; Karim, N.; Moez, B.; Oussama, J.; Hajer, N.; Habiba, B.S.A.; Zoukar, O.; Jemaa, Y. Acute acalculous cholecystitis in hospitalized patients in intensive care unit: Study of 5 cases. *Heliyon* **2022**, *8*, e11524. [CrossRef]
29. Whitcomb, D.C. Acute Pancreatitis [Internet]. 2013. Available online: https://pubmed.ncbi.nlm.nih.gov/16707751/ (accessed on 14 May 2023).
30. Almutairi, F.; Rabeie, N.; Awais, A.; Samannodi, M.; Aljehani, N.; Tayeb, S.; Elsayad, W. COVID-19 induced acute pancreatitis after resolution of the infection. *J. Infect. Public Health* **2022**, *15*, 282–284. [CrossRef]
31. Kumaran, N.K.; Karmakar, B.K.; Taylor, O.M. Coronavirus disease-19 (COVID-19) associated with acute necrotising pancreatitis (ANP). *BMJ Case Rep. CP* **2020**, *13*, e237903. [CrossRef]
32. Qian, D.H.; Zhu, G.J.; Wu, L.Z.; Hua, G.X. Isolation and characterization of a coronavirus from pigeons with pancreatitis. *Am. J. Vet. Res.* **2006**, *67*, 1575–1579. [CrossRef] [PubMed]
33. Samanta, J.; Gupta, R.; Singh, M.P.; Patnaik, I.; Kumar, A.; Kochhar, R. Coronavirus disease 2019 and the pancreas. *Pancreatology* **2020**, *20*, 1567–1575. [CrossRef] [PubMed]
34. Cheung, K.S.; Hung, I.F.N.; Chan, P.P.Y.; Lung, K.C.; Tso, E.; Liu, R.; Ng, Y.Y.; Chu, M.Y.; Chung, T.W.; Tam, A.R. Gastrointestinal Manifestations of SARS-CoV-2 Infection and Virus Load in Fecal Samples From a Hong Kong Cohort: Systematic Review and Meta-analysis. *Gastroenterology* **2020**, *159*, 81–95. [CrossRef] [PubMed]
35. Zippi, M.; Hong, W.; Traversa, G.; Maccioni, F.; De Biase, D.; Gallo, C.; Fiorino, S. Involvement of the exocrine pancreas during COVID-19 infection and possible pathogenetic hypothesis: A concise review Myc-mediated cell competition in cancer View project. *Infez. Med.* **2020**, *28*, 507–515. Available online: https://www.researchgate.net/publication/346609266 (accessed on 14 May 2023). [PubMed]
36. Abramczyk, U.; Nowaczyński, M.; Słomczyński, A.; Wojnicz, P.; Zatyka, P.; Kuzan, A. Consequences of COVID-19 for the Pancreas. *Int. J. Mol. Sci.* **2022**, *23*, 864. [CrossRef] [PubMed]
37. Sinagra, E.; Shahini, E.; Crispino, F.; Macaione, I.; Guarnotta, V.; Marasà, M.; Testai, S.; Pallio, S.; Albano, D.; Facciorusso, A.; et al. COVID-19 and the Pancreas: A Narrative Review. *Life* **2022**, *12*, 1292. [CrossRef] [PubMed]
38. Kumar, V.; Barkoudah, E.; Souza, D.A.T.; Jin, D.X.; McNabb-Baltar, J. Clinical course and outcome among patients with acute pancreatitis and COVID-19. *Eur. J. Gastroenterol. Hepatol.* **2021**, *33*, 695–700. [CrossRef]
39. Bircakova, B.; Bruha, R.; Lambert, L.; Grusova, G.; Michalek, P.; Burgetova, A. A bimodal pattern of the onset of COVID-19 related acute pancreatitis supports both the cytotoxic and immune-related pathogenesis—A systematic review. *Scand. J. Gastroenterol.* **2021**, *56*, 870–873. [CrossRef]
40. Mutneja, H.R.; Bhurwal, A.; Arora, S.; Goel, A.; Vohra, I.; Attar, B.M. Acute pancreatitis in patients with COVID-19 is more severe and lethal: A systematic review and meta-analysis. *Scand. J. Gastroenterol.* **2021**, *56*, 1467–1472. [CrossRef]
41. McKay, S.C.; Pathak, S.; Wilkin, R.J.W.; Kamarajah, S.K.; Wigmore, S.J.; Rees, J.; Dunne, D.F.; Garcea, G.; Ahmad, J.; de Liguori Carino, N.; et al. Impact of SARS-CoV-2 pandemic on pancreatic cancer services and treatment pathways: United Kingdom experience. *HPB* **2021**, *23*, 1656–1665. [CrossRef]
42. Conti, C.B.; Henchi, S.; Coppeta, G.P.; Testa, S.; Grassia, R. Bleeding in COVID-19 severe pneumonia: The other side of abnormal coagulation pattern? *Eur. J. Intern. Med.* **2020**, *77*, 147. [CrossRef] [PubMed]

43. De Roquetaillade, C.; Chousterman, B.G.; Tomasoni, D.; Zeitouni, M.; Houdart, E.; Guedon, A.; Reiner, P.; Bordier, R.; Gayat, E.; Montalescot, G.; et al. Unusual arterial thrombotic events in Covid-19 patients. *Int. J. Cardiol.* **2021**, *323*, 281–284. [CrossRef] [PubMed]
44. Js, A.; Sm, A.; Am, A.; Althobiani, M.; Rp, R.; Oyelade, T. Thoracic imaging outcomes in COVID-19 survivors. *World J. Radiol.* **2021**, *13*, 149–156.
45. Han, H.; Yang, L.; Liu, R.; Liu, F.; Liu, F.; Wu, K.L.; Li, J.; Liu, X.-H.; Zhu, C.-L. Prominent changes in blood coagulation of patients with SARS-CoV-2 infection. *Clin. Chem. Lab. Med.* **2020**, *58*, 1116–1120. [CrossRef] [PubMed]
46. Pessoa, M.S.L.; Lima, C.F.C.; Pimentel, A.C.F.; José Carlos Godeiro Costa, J.; Holanda, J.L.B. Multisystemic Infarctions in COVID-19: Focus on the Spleen. *Eur. J. Case Rep. Intern. Med.* **2020**, *7*, 001747. [CrossRef]
47. Ghafoor, S.; Germann, M.; Jüngst, C.; Müllhaupt, B.; Reiner, C.S.; Stocker, D. Imaging features of COVID-19-associated secondary sclerosing cholangitis on magnetic resonance cholangiopancreatography: A retrospective analysis. *Insights Imaging* **2022**, *13*, 128. [CrossRef]
48. Dane, B.; Smereka, P.; Wain, R.; Kim, D.; Katz, D.S. Hypercoagulability in Patients with Coronavirus Disease (COVID-19): Identification of Arterial and Venous Thromboembolism in the Abdomen, Pelvis, and Lower Extremities. *AJR Am. J. Roentgenol.* **2021**, *216*, 104–105. [CrossRef]
49. Hellinger, J.C.; Sirous, R.; Hellinger, R.L.; Krauthamer, A. Abdominal Presentation of COVID-19. *Appl. Radiol.* **2020**, *49*, 24–26. Available online: https://appliedradiology.com/articles/abdominal-presentation-of-covid-19 (accessed on 14 May 2023). [CrossRef]
50. Prasoppokakorn, T.; Kullavanijaya, P.; Pittayanon, R. Risk factors of active upper gastrointestinal bleeding in patients with COVID-19 infection and the effectiveness of PPI prophylaxis. *BMC Gastroenterol.* **2022**, *22*, 465. [CrossRef]
51. Özer, M.; Terzioğlu, S.G.; KeskinkılıçYağız, B.; Gürer, A.; Dinç, T.; Coşkun, A. Does COVID-19 increase the incidence of spontaneous rectus sheath hematoma? *Ulus. Travma Acil Cerrahi Derg.* **2022**, *28*, 920–926. [CrossRef]
52. Mackiewicz-Milewska, M.; Sakwińska, K.; Cisowska-Adamiak, M.; Szymkuć-Bukowska, I.; Ratuszek-Sadowska, D.; Mackiewicz-Nartowicz, H. Bleeding into the Abdominal and Ilio-Lumbar Muscles—A Rare Complication in the Course of COVID-19: Analysis of Four Cases and a Literature Review. *J. Clin. Med.* **2022**, *11*, 4712. [CrossRef] [PubMed]
53. Ashktorab, H.; Russo, T.; Oskrochi, G.; Latella, G.; Massironi, S.; Luca, M.; Chirumamilla, L.G.; Laiyemo, A.O.; Brim, H. Clinical and Endoscopic Outcomes in COVID-19 Patients with Gastrointestinal Bleeding. *Gastro Help Adv.* **2022**, *1*, 487–499. [CrossRef] [PubMed]
54. Martin, T.A.; Wan, D.W.; Hajifathalian, K.; Tewani, S.; Shah, S.L.; Mehta, A.; Kaplan, A.; Ghosh, G.; Choi, A.J.; Krisko, T.I.; et al. Gastrointestinal Bleeding in Patients With Coronavirus Disease 2019: A Matched Case-Control Study. *Am. J. Gastroenterol.* **2020**, *115*, 1609–1616. [CrossRef] [PubMed]
55. Mohamed, M.; Nassar, M.; Nso, N.; Alfishawy, M. Massive gastrointestinal bleeding in a patient with COVID-19. *Arab. J. Gastroenterol.* **2021**, *22*, 177. [CrossRef]
56. Abdelmohsen, M.A.; Alkandari, B.M.; Gupta, V.K.; Elsebaie, N. Gastrointestinal tract imaging findings in confirmed COVID-19 patients: A non-comparative observational study. *Egypt. J. Radiol. Nucl. Med.* **2021**, *52*, 52. [CrossRef]

Disclaimer/Publisher's Note: The statements, opinions and data contained in all publications are solely those of the individual author(s) and contributor(s) and not of MDPI and/or the editor(s). MDPI and/or the editor(s) disclaim responsibility for any injury to people or property resulting from any ideas, methods, instructions or products referred to in the content.

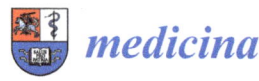

Review

Risk of New-Onset Liver Injuries Due to COVID-19 in Preexisting Hepatic Conditions—Review of the Literature

Sandica Bucurica [1,2], Florentina Ionita Radu [1,2,*], Ana Bucurica [1], Calin Socol [1], Ioana Prodan [1,2], Ioana Tudor [1,2], Carmen Adella Sirbu [3,4], Florentina Cristina Plesa [3,5,*] and Mariana Jinga [1,2]

1. Department of Gastroenterology, Carol Davila University of Medicine and Pharmacy, 020021 Bucharest, Romania
2. Department of Gastroenterology, 'Dr. Carol Davila' Central Military Emergency University Hospital, 010242 Bucharest, Romania
3. Department of Neurology, 'Dr. Carol Davila' Central Military Emergency University Hospital, 010242 Bucharest, Romania
4. Centre for Cognitive Research in Neuropsychiatric Pathology (Neuropsy-Cog), Department of Neurology, Faculty of Medicine, "Victor Babeș" University of Medicine and Pharmacy, 300041 Timișoara, Romania
5. Department of Preclinical Disciplines, Titu Maiorescu University of Medicine, 031593 Bucharest, Romania
* Correspondence: fionita04@yahoo.com (F.I.R.); plesacristina@yahoo.com (F.C.P.)

Abstract: The severe acute respiratory syndrome coronavirus 2 (SARS-CoV-2) impacted the world and caused the 2019 coronavirus disease (COVID-19) pandemic. The clinical manifestations of the virus can vary from patient to patient, depending on their respective immune system and comorbidities. SARS-CoV-2 can affect patients through two mechanisms: directly by targeting specific receptors or by systemic mechanisms. We reviewed data in the latest literature in order to discuss and determine the risk of new-onset liver injuries due to COVID-19 in preexisting hepatic conditions. The particular expression of angiotensin-converting enzyme 2 (ACE2) receptors is an additional risk factor for patients with liver disease. COVID-19 causes more severe forms in patients with non-alcoholic fatty liver disease (NAFLD), increases the risk of cirrhosis decompensation, and doubles the mortality for these patients. The coinfection SARS-CoV-2—viral hepatitis B or C might have different outcomes depending on the stage of the liver disease. Furthermore, the immunosuppressant treatment administered for COVID-19 might reactivate the hepatic virus. The high affinity of SARS-CoV-2 spike proteins for cholangiocytes results in a particular type of secondary sclerosing cholangitis. The impact of COVID-19 infection on chronic liver disease patients is significant, especially in cirrhosis, influencing the prognosis and outcome of these patients.

Keywords: liver cirrhosis; SARS-CoV-2; COVID-19; hepatitis; cholangitis; chronic liver disease

1. Introduction

Coronavirus disease 2019 (COVID-19), caused by infection with the severe acute respiratory syndrome coronavirus 2 (SARS-CoV-2), can affect people of any age and medical history, but it is known that patients with associated comorbidities have a higher risk of developing a more severe form of the disease [1].

The cumulative number of COVID-19 reached more than 604 million confirmed cases, with over 6.4 million deaths, according to published data in September 2022 [2].

SARS-CoV-2 infection may have different clinical manifestations, from asymptomatic to mild forms or severe multisystem involvement [3,4].

In 2021, it was estimated that approximately 1.5 billion patients worldwide suffered from chronic liver disease [5]. The World Health Organization (WHO) estimated in 2019 that 296 million people worldwide were living with hepatitis B and 58 million with hepatitis C, and that almost 1.5 million people for each type are newly infected every year [6,7]. The

---

Citation: Bucurica, S.; Ionita Radu, F.; Bucurica, A.; Socol, C.; Prodan, I.; Tudor, I.; Sirbu, C.A.; Plesa, F.C.; Jinga, M. Risk of New-Onset Liver Injuries Due to COVID-19 in Preexisting Hepatic Conditions—Review of the Literature. *Medicina* 2023, *59*, 62. https://doi.org/10.3390/medicina59010062

Academic Editor: Daniel Paramythiotis and Eleni Karlafti

Received: 30 November 2022
Revised: 21 December 2022
Accepted: 23 December 2022
Published: 28 December 2022

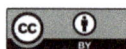

Copyright: © 2022 by the authors. Licensee MDPI, Basel, Switzerland. This article is an open access article distributed under the terms and conditions of the Creative Commons Attribution (CC BY) license (https:// creativecommons.org/licenses/by/ 4.0/).

prevalence of non-alcoholic fatty liver disease (NAFLD) is constantly increasing, matching the rise in the prevalence of obesity [8].

Regarding liver dysfunction during COVID-19, although not all pathways are clear, it has been shown that up to 50% of patients have altered liver enzymes and hepatic impairment [4,9].

Pathophysiologically, SARS-CoV-2 has a direct cytopathic action, binding to the angiotensin-convertase 2 (ACE2) receptors, abundantly expressed in hepatic and biliary epithelial cells.

Histological studies found a variety of liver alterations: slight infiltration of lymphocytes in lobuli associated with a degree of dilation or thrombosis in centrilobular sinusoids, portal inflammation or calcification [10], and variable steatosis degrees going up to the fibrotic stage [11].

Vascular abnormalities and necrosis have been described in a number of studies, which are determined by venous endoluminal obstruction, lymphocytic endotheliosis, and hypoperfusion [12,13]. Fractions of the novel corona virus were identified in hepatic cytoplasm [14], and viral specific proteins were detected in cholangiocytes [15] and hepatocytes even half a year after infection [16].

The affinity of the SARS-CoV-2 virus for cholangiocytes and the biliary tract is high. The viral particles were also present in the gallbladder [17], and congestive alterations with a micro-thrombotic vascular pattern, congestion, and gallbladder mucosa friability were found, similar to SARS-CoV-2 hepatic damage [18].

From an immunological perspective, the relationship between the liver and SARS-CoV-2 is complex and combines the tissue direct viral action with the systemic pro-inflammatory response and "cytokine storm" [19].

ACE-2 receptors (ACE-2R), which are abundant in cholangiocytes and in the cells of the sinusoid endothelium and fewer in the hepatic cells [20], and trans-membrane protease serine 2 (TMPRSS2) are the two most important elements that contribute to SARS-CoV-2 infectiveness [21].

The virus can use an alternative pathway—furin, a protein convertase—to gain access to the host cells. The viral structure is composed of nucleocapsid (N), membrane, envelope, and spike proteins (S) [22]. As a result, the virion spike protein S can bind to the ACE 2 receptors and TMPRSS2 or use furin proteinase cleaving action.

The inflammatory and immune systemic response in SARS-CoV-2 infection is mediated by the breakdown of T cell lymphocytes, flare of interleukin 6 (IL-6), and tumor necrosis factor-α (TNF-α). The complement overstimulation pathway appears to be another mechanism that leads to hyperinflammation through the IFN-Janus kinase (JAK) 1/2-signal transducer and activator of transcription (STAT) signaling complex alongside nuclear factor kappa B (NF-kB) [23,24].

Acute liver injury (ALI) during systemic inflammation caused by COVID-19 corresponds to increased c-reactive protein (CRP) levels, elevated interleukin-6, and high ferritin [25]. Pro-thrombotic status induced by SARS-CoV-2 contributes to liver affliction through vessel endothelial injury, intravascular emboli, micro/macro thrombosis induced by immune dysregulation, platelet impairment, and hypoxemia [26].

Hepatic injury in COVID-19 patients can be assessed using liver biochemical tests: serum albumin, cholestasis markers-bilirubin, gamma-glutamyl transferase (GGT), alkaline phosphatase (ALP), liver transaminases-aspartate aminotransferase (AST/TGO), and alanine aminotransferase (ALT/TGP) [27,28]. A larger study found ALT and AST to be more than 3x the upper limit of normal (ULN) and bilirubin more than 2x ULN in patients with severe COVID-19, and AST to be higher than ALT, which can be a consequence of immune-mediated inflammation or injury [27,29].

The data presented by another study with more than 1000 patients showed AST serum values 3 times higher in patients with severe COVID-19 compared to those with the mild form of the disease [29,30]. It was observed that AST levels rise early in the disease course, and AST is more elevated than ALT [31,32].

One Chinese study published in 2021 evaluated serum albumin as a possible predictor for COVID-19 outcome [33]. Hypoalbuminemia was frequently found in infected patients, especially those with severe forms. Moreover, the level of albumin was correlated with the magnitude of the inflammatory status (lymphocyte, total number of T cells–CD4 and CD8, hemoglobin levels, and red blood cell numbers), but was not associated with CRP and AST [34]. Hypoalbuminemia is not a result of reduced synthesis in severe COVID-19, but a result of albumin consumption [35]. One study revealed that SARS-CoV-2 needs and utilizes albumin, so immediate albumin therapy is recommended for severe COVID-19 [36].

When it comes to the role of gamma-glutamyl transpeptidase (GGT) in COVID-19, it was found that increased GGT and AST are directly proportional to longer hospitalization. A study established an association between GGT and the expression of ACE2 connected to the common transcriptional hepatic nuclear factor-1β (HNF1B), which points out the possibility of using GGT as a biomarker for SARS-CoV-2 susceptibility [37]. A retrospective clinical study of 98 patients hospitalized at Wenzhou Central Hospital in Wenzhou, China, from January to February 2020, showed that 32.7% presented elevated GGT levels and 22.5% had increased CRP [38]. Moreover, a study that followed 118 COVID-19 patients for 376 days highlighted that elevated ALT, AST GGT, and body mass index (BMI) immediately after hospitalization were still increased 1 year after discharge, which emphasizes the need for close monitoring of patients with liver abnormalities [39].

2. Materials and Methods

The main purpose of this review was to establish, from the latest published data, the impact of COVID-19 infection on preexisting liver conditions.

We searched the databases PubMed, National Library of Medicine, the World Health Organization International Clinical Trials Registry Platform (ICTRP), the World Health Organization International Clinical Trials Registry Platform (ICTRP), Google Scholar, and Google during the pandemic era, starting from the beginning of 2020, until now, September 2022, for articles written, especially, in English that described the effects of COVID-19 infection on preexisting liver conditions. The search was carried out using the search terms "coronavirus", "COVID-19", and "SARS-CoV-2", combined with "liver", "hepatic", "cirrhosis", "NAFLD", "hepatitis", "liver tests", "cholangitis", and "inflammation".

Research articles, reviews, case series, and case reports were taken into consideration, and almost all of the 123 articles cited were analyzed further. We excluded articles that included hepatocellular carcinoma, as any alteration in this stage can influence the course of the disease. Drug-induced liver injury (DILI) articles were excluded. The multitude of DILI can be a separate article because of the large number of medications used to treat COVID-19 infection with possible hepatic alterations that may overlap with the drugs used in preexisting liver diseases.

We paid attention to articles connected to liver injuries provoked only by COVID-19 but with no further evaluation.

The secondary sclerosing cholangitis determined by COVID-19 was included even though it is related to the cholestatic effect of COVID-19, and only case series and case reports were found.

3. COVID-19 and Cirrhosis

Cirrhosis is the final stage of long-term liver disease, causing an alteration in liver architecture through processes such as the production of extensive nodules, neo-angiogenesis, vascular restructuring, and newly formed extracellular matrix deposits [40]. Chronic liver disease is characterized by a cyclic process consisting of inflammation leading to the destruction and subsequent regeneration of liver parenchyma [40]. Cirrhosis may develop as a consequence of this process over the years, but at the time the diagnosis is made, it is considered irreversible [40]. Chronic liver disease causes immune dysregulation and inflammation, which can have an augmented effect on the processes present in SARS-CoV-2 infection [41].

The expression of ACE2 in hepatocytes of cirrhotic patients is 30 times higher than in the normal liver, and the association of metabolic syndrome increases the expression of both ACE2 and TMPRSS2 [42].

COVID-19 might affect the liver directly [43] (hepatocyte destruction caused directly by the SARS-CoV-2 virus or through viral translocation from the gut to the liver) or by indirect mechanisms [43] (such as systemic inflammation, hypoxemic effects on preexisting liver diseases, or ICU admission length) [43].

SARS-CoV-2 infection and cirrhosis seem to be a fatal combination, with augmented immune dysregulation being at the core of further biological processes leading to a more severe form of the disease [41]. Inflammation, in this case, is predominantly initiated by circulating active immune cells and pro-inflammatory cytokines [44].

One study estimated the overall mortality in patients with cirrhosis and SARS-CoV-2 association at about 32%, the mortality and morbidity increasing for patients with a higher Child-Pugh score, a widely used tool to assess the prognosis of patients with cirrhosis [44]. In this study, Child-Pugh class C patients had a 21% survival chance if admitted to the intensive care unit (ICU), dropping to 10% if they were on mechanical ventilation [45]. Another study revealed that mortality is also influenced by different risk factors such as advanced age, obesity, type II diabetes (T2D) or cardiovascular diseases; 78.7% of COVID-19 patients had lung-related conditions as the cause of death, while 4.3% of deaths were caused by cardiovascular disease and 12.2% by liver conditions [45].

The results from the COVID-Hep registry data showed that patients with fibrotic stage liver disease have a higher death rate [44]. This analysis included 745 patients, 386 with cirrhosis, showing a 32% mortality in this group, which is 4 times higher compared with non-cirrhotic ones, with an overall mortality of 20% (150 deaths/745 patients) [44]. The risk factors were higher Child-Pugh scores (C vs. A—51% vs. 19%), age, being Caucasian (OR 2.52; 95% CI 1.73–3.68; $p < 0.001$), cardiovascular comorbidities, and renal function impairment (OR 1.19 per mg/dl; 95% CI 1.04–1.38; $p = 0.014$) [44].

Moreover, another study confirmed that the Child-Pugh class can be used to assess the prognosis of SARS-CoV-2 infection by determining the risk of decompensation—64% for the C class compared to 30% for the Child-Pugh A class [46]. It presented as ascites or aggravation of the current ascites in 109 patients (28%), portal encephalopathy, rupture of varices in 27% of cases, and 3% with spontaneous bacterial peritonitis [46].

The death rates for patients with fibrotic stage liver disease were evaluated in large studies worldwide, and a mortality between 25 and 51% was found for cirrhotic patients with SARS-CoV-2 infection [47,48]. The mortality was lower in patients with compensated forms versus decompensated forms, 14% vs. 40.8% (n = 19/134 and n = 38/93) [49].

Invasive ventilation was necessary in 24% of the cases with decompensated cirrhosis, compared with 19% in patients with compensated forms [50].

One study from northern Europe found no clear link between COVID-19 and the outcome or evolution of cirrhosis [51]. A meta-analysis that focused on the outcome of COVID-19 infection in cirrhotic and non-cirrhotic patients included 40 studies with more than 900,000 participants. This showed that the COVID-19-cirrhosis association had an increased risk for severity (OR = 2.44; 95% CI, 1.89–3.16) and death (OR = 2.35; 95% CI, 1.85–3.00) [52].

The symptomatology of COVID-19 infection in cirrhotic patients has a specific course. First, acute decompensation is found in 46% of the patients, with formation or worsening of ascites and/or the onset of hepatic encephalopathy. In total, 20–58% of patients can present these alterations without respiratory symptoms connected to COVID-19 [44].

Gastrointestinal manifestations are another possible presentation for these patients, and they are thought to be connected to increased gut permeability, electrolytic changes, and systemic inflammation [49].

A series of severity scoring classifications can be used to assess the cirrhotic patients' status, showing poorer prognosis for patients with cirrhosis and COVID-19 compared with non-COVID-19 patients [53,54].

A study from India found increased mortality for patients with acute-on-chronic liver failure (ACLF) [55]. The mortality rate of patients with ACLF–COVID-19 association was 55% [54].

ACE2 internalization by SARS-CoV-2 causes reduced ACE2 activity with further alteration in the pathway of angiotensin-II. The role of angiotensin-II in the renin-angiotensin system is essential for vasoconstriction, renal sodium retention, and promoting hepatic fibrogenesis. The reduced number of ACE2 in cirrhotic patients with COVID-19 aggravates hepatic fibrosis and portal hypertension, exacerbating the severity of the disease [56–58].

The interaction between SARS-CoV-2 and the liver appears to be a vicious circle, ultimately leading to multiple system organ failure (MSOF) [59]. Another study showed that COVID-19 was found to increase by 5-fold the chance of death among cirrhotic patients, respectively accounting for a 2.2-fold increase in the death risk of those with decompensated cirrhosis [46,60], but the main cause of death in cirrhotic patients infected with COVID-19 was found to be respiratory failure (71% of the cases in the study), while only 19% of the patients died of complications related to the liver [61].

4. COVID-19 and Cholangitis

Secondary sclerosing cholangitis is a progressive disease defined by intense fibrosis and destruction of the biliary tract, which can lead to biliary cirrhosis. Secondary sclerosis cholangitis in critically ill patients (SSC-CIP) is a form of secondary cholangiopathy that can cause a rapid deterioration of the patients [61,62].

Cholestasis in critically ill patients is mostly intrahepatic and is a result of the complex pathology behind it, such as systemic inflammatory response syndrome (SIRS), ischemic hepatitis, drug-induced liver injury, parenteral support, and ventilatory support [63]. A cholestatic pattern is less frequent in acute COVID-19 infection [61].

Secondary sclerosis cholangitis in critically ill patients (SSC-CIP) caused by SARS-CoV-2 was defined as a cholestatic liver injury that develops post-COVID-19 infection [64].

Despite emerging reports of secondary sclerosing cholangitis (SSC) in critically ill SARS-CoV-2-infected patients, there are no specific imagistic features that could be associated with the evolution of delayed progressive cholestatic liver injury, leading to cirrhosis [64].

Anatomically, the biliary system receives blood only from the peribiliary vascular plexus, while the liver parenchyma has two major blood supplies. The hypothesis of ischemia has been used to explain that severe hypotension with decreased mean arterial pressure (MAP) and longer time spent in the prone position are the triggers of SSC-CIP [65]. The incidence of SSC-CIP is directly proportional to ICU stay, even in patients without any history of biliary or liver disease. SSC-CIP is defined as a significant complication of ICU stay [66].

This new variant of sclerosis cholangitis provoked by COVID-19 is characterized by liver enzyme elevation even in patients who have not been to the ICU [67]. Pathologists have reported that severe cholangitic injury and intrahepatic microangiopathy are found in COVID-19 infection [67]. When comparing the level of RNA between airway cells and hepatic cells, there is a similar range but a lower median viral RNA in hepatic cells [68].

The binding of SARS-CoV-2 to the ACE2-R from cholangiocytes affects the barrier and the mechanism of transportation of the bile acid by affecting gene regulation. This leads to cholestasis and liver damage [69,70].

A retrospective study conducted in one center in Zurich on 34 patients admitted with COVID-19 to the ICU showed that 14 (41%) had mild cholestasis and 9 (27%) presented with a severe form of cholestasis [63]. Moreover, the ICU stay was prolonged for the last group of patients, and 4 of them developed secondary sclerosing cholangitis [63].

One study showed the case of a 38-year-old male with COVID-19 pneumonia that developed, afterward, hyperbilirubinemia, jaundice, and elevated transaminases [71]. He was hospitalized multiple times for pain, nausea, vomiting, and elevated liver enzymes, which resolved with supportive treatment. The patient underwent magnetic resonance cholangiopancreatography (MRCP), which revealed diffuse intrahepatic biliary distention and irregularity in the extrahepatic common bile duct. After performing the biopsy (cholangiocyte injury, bile ductular proliferation, canalicular cholestasis, fibrosis), the diagnosis of secondary sclerosing cholangitis was taken into consideration [71].

Biliary damage in COVID-19 patients should be taken into consideration when clinical and biological findings reveal jaundice, elevated transaminases, and/or cholestasis. Biliary imaging should be performed to confirm/infirm SSC [71].

One study that enrolled 496 patients showed that 15.4% of patients developed SSC, and patients with both chronic liver disease and COVID-19 pneumonia had a higher risk [72].

The multisystemic effect of SARS-CoV-2 has been intensively studied. The connection between COVID-19 and SSC was underlined, as several case reports have been published [73]. A middle-aged man came to the emergency room after being infected with SARS-CoV-2, with aggravating jaundice, abdominal pain, elevated liver enzymes, and dark-colored urine [73]. He underwent endoscopic retrograde cholangiopancreatography (ERCP) and MRCP, and the diagnosis of SSC was established based on the findings; he was registered for liver transplantation [73].

Another study presented chronic cholestasis and liver injury developed after COVID-19 [74]. Histopathologically, cholangiocyte injury with microvascular changes was observed. In one case, fibrosis and the presence of cytokeratin 7 metaplasia of periportal hepatocytes (an important factor for obstructive cholestasis) were reported [74].

A study presented the case of a patient who continued to have chronic cholestasis and liver injury after severe sepsis connected to COVID-19 [75]. The diagnosis of SSC was established after a liver biopsy, and ursodiol 250 mg three times a day was administered. After 6 months, the patient was discharged, and jaundice and elevated liver enzymes were ameliorated, but still persistently elevated [75].

One study published this year compared 24 patients with SSC after COVID-19 with 77 patients with SSC-CIP [66]. The median for SSC development was 91 days after COVID-19. There were no differences in most of the symptoms and transplant-free survival. Ursodeoxycholic acid treatment and albumin were administered [66]. Even though there are similarities between these two entities, the authors concluded that the course of the disease and the risk factors are unrelated between the two pathologies, and ursodeoxycholic acid administration needs further validation [66].

There is no established protocol for SSC treatment, and the last curative option is liver transplantation [76,77].

5. COVID-19 and NAFLD (Non-Alcoholic Fatty Liver Disease)

Non-alcoholic fatty liver disease (NAFLD) is defined as hepatic steatosis with or without inflammation and/or fibrosis [78]. The disease is further divided into NAFL—non-alcoholic fatty liver (NAFL) and non-alcoholic steatohepatitis (NASH), the main difference between them being the presence of inflammation [78]. Liver biopsy is the gold standard method of diagnosing NAFLD (staging from milder forms (steatosis) to severe forms (NASH, advanced fibrosis, cirrhosis)). Histologically, NAFLD has been defined as the presence of hepatic steatosis, ballooning, and lobular inflammation with or without fibrosis [79].

NAFLD is a heterogenous condition, mainly related to the types of lipids that accumulate, their toxicity to the liver, and to the ability of the individual to defend against it. The response of wound healing of individuals determines their capacity to recover from NASH or to develop scarring, cirrhosis, and even hepatocellular carcinoma [79].

NAFLD is becoming a leading cause of chronic liver disease worldwide because of the high incidence of both obesity and metabolic syndrome [80].

While the prevalence of the disease varies with age, sex, and demographics, it is more common in Hispano-American men aged between 40 and 50 years [78].

A systematic review revealed that COVID-19 infection has a more severe course in NAFLD patients, being correlated to ICU stay [81]. Furthermore, NAFLD is a significant risk factor for COVID-19, a finding that has been further proven accurate after the adjustment was made for obesity as a confounding factor [82]. Controversially, a few articles have stated that NAFLD does not influence the rate of mortality [83,84] or the outcome of COVID-19 [83,85]. NAFLD can be a predictor of consecutive hepatic injuries [85]. Although NAFLD might not be a major risk factor for a worse outcome in COVID-19, those patients often have other associated pathologies that may influence the course of the disease (e.g., metabolic syndrome) [61].

A case-control study in 2021 evaluated 71 patients divided into two groups: with or without fatty liver on CT scans. In total, 22 (31%) had NAFLD [86]. Severe forms of COVID-19 developed in NAFLD patients ($p < 0.005$), providing further evidence for NAFLD as a risk factor for a poor prognosis [86].

Another study confirmed that the risk for hospitalization and severity is higher in patients with NAFLD/NASH regardless of gender or race [87]. Moreover, after receiving treatment for NAFLD/NASH, obese patients have a diminished risk for hospitalization [87].

Patients with NAFLD (particularly those with NASH) often have one or more components of metabolic syndrome, to which NAFLD is linked [88]. SARS-CoV-2 infection is known to have a worse outcome in patients with high BMI or diabetes [89]. The pathophysiological mechanism is related to obesity-related poor immune responses to infection. It has been postulated that there is chronic inflammation in obese patients with pro-inflammatory citokine release mediated by the NLRP3 inflammasome [89].

NAFLD is not only associated with COVID-19, but it can increase the risk of developing all types of infections through systemic alterations, such as hyperglycemia, insulin resistance, alteration of innate immunity, obesity, and vitamin D deficiency [90].

The lockdown caused changes in lifestyle: more coffee and tobacco use and less physical activity [91]. Moreover, during the pandemic era, NAFLD and insulin resistance prevalence worsened as a consequence of the lack of screening and regular monitoring of patients [91].

Research related to fatty liver index was published evaluating 3122 COVID-19 patients from the South Korea database [92]. The aim was to correlate the fatty liver index (FLI) of NAFLD patients with the severity of COVID-19, showing that NAFLD patients have a poorer prognosis and a higher likelihood of needing mechanical ventilation, ICU admission, and high flow oxygen therapy. As a result, FLI can be used to assess the prognosis of COVID-19 [92].

SARS-CoV-2 infection increases the likelihood of developing new types of liver dysfunctions [88]. The majority of the macrophages are hosted in the liver, and as the macrophages have an impeded clearance in the SARS-CoV-2 infection, it leads to further alteration of liver function through augmented cytokine production [88]. In NAFLD patients, the polarization status of macrophages might be affected, influencing the inflammatory response to SARS-CoV-2. A study conducted in central London concluded that there was no statistically significant difference regarding mortality or ICU admissions between patients with NAFLD and those without. The main difference was that patients with NAFLD were younger and had a higher inflammatory response at the time of admission [83].

Excessive weight and NAFLD associate a pro-inflammatory status with high levels of pro-inflammatory cytokines [93] (NLR family pyrin domain containing 3—NLPR3, IL-1 [89]), increasing susceptibility to severe infection. Obese patients with NASH have a higher risk of being infected with COVID-19, as they have higher liver mRNA expression of ACE2 and TMMPRS 2 [94].

NAFLD is frequently present in patients with metabolic syndrome (hyperglycemic syndrome, hypertriglyceridemia, hypertension, raised high-density lipoprotein cholesterol HDL-cholesterol, obesity), and the influence of ACE2-R has been studied in patients with NAFLD and in those with type 2 diabetes [94]. In T2D, it was observed that there are lower amounts of ACE2-R in comparison to TMPRSS2, which showed no statistically significant difference. Furthermore, ACE2-R is more present in men with T2D than in women. We can theorize, based on the available data, that the main mechanism of the entrance of

SARS-CoV-2 is not majorly altered in the livers of obese men with T2D, but there may be a lower susceptibility for liver injury in women [94].

COVID-19 enters the cholangiocytes through ACE2-R and causes direct damage with liver enzyme alteration, including albumin, GGT, ALT, and AST [95–97]. Moreover, the cytokine storm activated in COVID-19 affects the liver directly. TNF-α, a pro-inflammatory protein, is produced by adipose tissue and liver macrophages and modifies the immune response in patients with NAFLD. This process has consequences for M1 macrophages, which are suppressed, while M2 macrophages have an intense activation [95–97]. Taking this statement into account, it is necessary to identify a targeted treatment to reduce FLI [95–97].

A recent study attempted to find a connection between COVID-19 chronic sequelae and the progression to NAFLD [98]. The hypothesis was that systemic inflammation, all metabolic changes, including changes in the gut microbiome, and stimulation of liver fibrosis can be caused by COVID-19 [98]. A trend for liver enzyme alteration, steatosis, hyperplasia of Kupffer cells, and hepatobiliary congestion was revealed. The liver was indirectly affected, as the main targets were the ACE2-R [98]. The release of pro-inflammatory cytokines might trigger NASH development through their systemic effect [98]. Changes in the gut microbiome have been observed in a large number of patients with COVID-19 [98,99], but further studies are needed.

6. COVID-19 and Hepatitis B and C Infection

Hepatitis represents the inflammation of the liver caused by a variety of factors, frequently hepatic viruses (A, B, C, D, E). Diagnosis can be made by testing the presence of specific antiviral antigens or antibodies. Hepatitis B is caused by an enveloped virus containing an incomplete double-stranded, circular DNA genome [100]. It has different clinical outcomes depending on the patient's status (age, immune status, or stage of the disease) [100].

Another infection is hepatitis C, which nowadays is the major cause of cirrhosis and hepatocarcinoma. It became curable with treatment development, which can lead to eradication in 98% of infected patients [101,102].

Moreover, because viral hepatic infections are a public health issue, the WHO is attempting to eradicate them by 2030 through an intense surveillance program of infected patients, accurate treatment, or vaccination [103,104].

A clinical study suggests that either current or past infection with HBV does not influence the risk of severe liver injury in SARS-CoV-2 coinfection [105].

In a large study that included SARS-CoV-2 infected patients (675 with HBV infection and 18,485 patients without signs of infection), it was observed that HBV-positive patients were older and more frail than HBV-negative ones. The COVID-19 mortality rate was evaluated at 8.2% in the HBV-negative group and 13.5% in the HBV-positive group. Moreover, COVID-19 and HBV-positive patients required intensive care unit admission and had a higher risk of MSOF [106]. In this study, it was concluded that COVID-19 and HBV infection influence the survival rate of the patients [106]. Using antiviral therapies might provide a higher risk of progression to liver failure but might reduce the risk of respiratory insufficiency [106].

Treatment for COVID-19 implies one agent that works against the SARS-CoV-2 virus itself or one against the inflammatory response of the host [105].

Liver injury in COVID-19 patients can be attributed to direct viral effects on the liver and/or hepatotoxic drugs, as proven by the elevated liver enzymes found in these patients [107,108]. The viral HBV reactivation after monoclonal antibodies (tocilizumab) and corticosteroid usage raises the need for careful screening before prescription [107,108].

The prognosis of infection with SARS-CoV-2 in HBV patients depends on the stage of liver disease, as proposed by Shanshan Yang et al. [109]. Therefore, HBV infection with HBeAg (+) can cause a bad outcome for patients compared to infection with HBeAg (−) [109]. Moreover, age is essential for the prognosis of HBeAg (+) VHB infection and for HBV reactivation [109]. Moreover, a great number of these patients presented with abnormal liver function and severe status requiring ICU admission [109].

Chen et al. observed that there are no differences in hospital length of stay between HBV-positive and HBV-negative coinfected patients [110]. He et al. observed the same aspect and also showed that coinfection is not associated with a poorer prognosis [111].

On the other hand, another study observed that patients who have a hepatic infection during the coinfection stage have a higher liver alteration. A multicentric study from Wuhan, China, observed that abnormal AST or DBIL levels are not risk factors for COVID-19 mortality, but they can be considered independent risk factors [112].

A study published in the *American Journal of Gastroenterology* reported that HBV incidence among patients with SARS-CoV-2 infection was lower compared with the overall incidence of HBV infection in the Chinese population [113]. It has been theorized that the excess of T lymphocytes can affect the ability of these patients to respond to other viruses so that the cytokine storm is reduced and the severity of COVID-19 is decreased [113].

During the pandemic, the number of hepatitis C virus RNA tests decreased by 62% in March 2020 and remained at 39%, below the baseline, by July 2020 [114]. When it comes to hepatitis C and COVID-19, the use of immunosuppressants is associated with a risk of HCV reactivation [115,116].

The two pathophysiological mechanisms involved are the stimulation of viral replication, directly, and the suppression of the immune system [117]. These two mechanisms might cause HCV reactivation [117]. Moreover, HCV viremia increases during corticosteroid treatment and can return to the baseline when the medication is discontinued [117].

Having a history of HCV infection might make a patient more susceptible to severe respiratory complications, without the influence of any other comorbidity, a biological marker at admission, or COVID-19 liver injury [118]. The effect seems to be correlated to the extrahepatic effects of HCV, stimulating ACE-2/TMPRSS mechanisms, the inflammatory process, and endothelial dysfunction [119].

A multicenter retrospective study evaluated 125 patients with chronic hepatitis and COVID-19 (64 patients with cirrhosis). They presented with a large variety of symptoms, but cough, core throat, fatigue, myalgia, and diarrhea were more frequent in cirrhotic patients. They discovered many independent factors that can influence the outcome of patients: male gender, diabetes mellitus, and cirrhosis [118].

When the HCV and COVID-19 coinfection was evaluated for the inflammatory response and the cytokine types involved, the levels of interleukin 17 and 6 were found to be higher in coinfected patients compared with patients infected only with SARS-CoV-2 [120].

Sofosbuvir, tenofovir, and ribavirin, an antiviral treatment used for HBV and HCV, have been shown to have activity against infected patients with SARS-CoV-2 through their binding to the RNA-dependent-RNA polymerase (RdRp) of the coronavirus [121], but future trials are needed.

Furthermore, a form of transient hepatitis in a patient that tested positive for the SARS-CoV-2 virus, named COVID-19-induced hepatitis (CIH), was described. It might progress with elevated ALT and AST, non-obstructive jaundice, and inflammatory infiltration of the liver parenchyma [122]. An increased AST/ALT ratio is linked to systemic inflammation, while a low ratio is related to liver injury [123].

With ongoing research about COVID-19 and its connection with liver alteration going on, an isoquinoline alkaloid, called berberine, was found to have important activity against COVID-19, with multiple effects—antiviral, anti-allergy, and anti-inflammatory—ensuring hepatoprotection against drugs and infection-induced liver injury while reducing oxidative stress [124]. Berberine can have an antiviral effect against various agents (influenza, hepatitis B, hepatitis C, cytomegalovirus, alphavirus, and papillomavirus) [124]. The mechanism of this agent is still under evaluation, but it is clear that it can increase IFN-γ levels by intense stimulation of CD8 T cells and can inhibit histamine release from mast cells. Moreover, ACE2, IL-1α, IL-8, IL-6, and chemokine ligand 2 (CCL-2) are inhibited by berberine administration. It can be beneficial not only for COVID-19 treatment but also for viral infection treatment or eradication [124].

One study proved that berberine has a beneficial role in treating the bacterial infections associated with COVID-19 and in reducing hydroxychloroquine toxicity [125].

Berberine can be a promising treatment for hepatic C infection. It has been found to affect the entry/fusion into the cell of the virus. Moreover, it inhibits viral pseudoparticles E1/E2 [126,127]. It might become a possible antiviral treatment for HBV infection because of its effect on mitogen-activated protein kinase (MAPK) pathways. Kim et al. suggested that berberine acts like a p38 MAPK inhibitor and, in this way, can cause HBsAg suppression [127,128].

Another promising molecule is 8-hydroxydihydrosanguinarine, a phyto-alkaloid that interferes in the connection of S protein to ACE2, which indicates a potential therapy for COVID-19 [129], but further studies are needed.

7. Conclusions

The systemic inflammation developed during COVID-19 may change the course of hepatic preexisting diseases, with additional morphofunctional alterations of the liver, and may cause a persistent effect from that point forward.

The impact of COVID-19 infection on cirrhotic patients is significant, influencing their prognosis and outcome. Medical societies have raised awareness about the exposure of these patients.

There are premises of a new emerging entity caused by the SARS-CoV-2 virus—the secondary sclerosis cholangitis in critically ill patients, without any preexisting liver conditions.

The polymerization used to treat SARS-CoV-2 infection is continuously changing, exposing the patients with preexisting liver alterations to more and more possible complications.

The effects of COVID-19 on the liver are a challenge for doctors, raising concern about the medical approach and treatment of patients with preexisting hepatic conditions.

Author Contributions: Conceptualization, S.B. and I.P.; resources, A.B., C.S. and F.C.P.; writing—original draft preparation, I.P.; writing—review and editing, S.B. and I.P.; supervision, C.A.S., I.T., M.J. and F.I.R. All authors have read and agreed to the published version of the manuscript.

Funding: This paper was partially supported by "Carol Davila" University of Medicine and Pharmacy Bucharest, Romania through Contract no. 33PFE/30.12.2021 funded by the Ministry of Research and Innovation within PNCDI III, Program 1-Development of the National RD system, Subprogram 1.2-Institutional Performance-RDI excellence funding projects.

Institutional Review Board Statement: Not applicable.

Informed Consent Statement: Not applicable.

Data Availability Statement: Not applicable.

Conflicts of Interest: The authors declare no conflict of interest.

References

1. Sanyaolu, A.; Okorie, C.; Marinkovic, A.; Patidar, R.; Younis, K.; Desai, P.; Hosein, Z.; Padda, I.; Mangat, J.; Altaf, M. Comorbidity and its Impact on Patients with COVID-19. *SN Compr. Clin. Med.* **2020**, *2*, 1069–1076. [CrossRef] [PubMed]
2. WHO Coronavirus (COVID-19) Dashboard. Available online: https://covid19.who.int (accessed on 9 October 2022).
3. Heydari, K.; Lotfi, P.; Shadmehri, N.; Yousefi, M.; Raei, M.; Houshmand, P.; Zahedi, M.; Alizadeh-Navaei, R.; Bathaeian, S.; Rismantab, S. Clinical and Paraclinical Characteristics of COVID-19 patients: A Systematic Review and Meta-Analysis. *Tabari Biomed. Stud. Res. J.* **2022**, *4*, 30–47. [CrossRef]
4. Zahedi, M.; Yousefi, M.; Abounoori, M.; Malekan, M.; Tajik, F.; Heydari, K.; Mortazavi, P.; Ghahramani, S.; Ghazaeian, M.; Sheydaee, F.; et al. The Interrelationship between Liver Function Test and the Coronavirus Disease 2019: A Systematic Review and Meta-Analysis. *Iran. J. Med. Sci.* **2021**, *46*, 237–255. [CrossRef] [PubMed]
5. Cheemerla, S.; Balakrishnan, M. Global Epidemiology of Chronic Liver Disease. *Clin. Liver Dis.* **2021**, *17*, 365–370. [CrossRef] [PubMed]
6. Global Progress Report on HIV, Viral Hepatitis and Sexually Transmitted Infections. 2021. Available online: https://www.who.int/publications-detail-redirect/9789240027077 (accessed on 9 October 2022).

7. Hepatitis, C. Available online: https://www.who.int/news-room/fact-sheets/detail/hepatitis-c (accessed on 9 October 2022).
8. Vernon, G.; Baranova, A.; Younossi, Z.M. Systematic review: The epidemiology and natural history of non-alcoholic fatty liver disease and non-alcoholic steatohepatitis in adults. *Aliment. Pharmacol. Ther.* **2011**, *34*, 274–285. [CrossRef] [PubMed]
9. Chen, T.; Wu, D.; Chen, H.; Yan, W.; Yang, D.; Chen, G.; Ma, K.; Xu, D.; Yu, H.; Wang, H.; et al. Clinical characteristics of 113 deceased patients with coronavirus disease 2019: Retrospective study. *BMJ* **2020**, *368*, m1091. [CrossRef]
10. Tian, S.; Xiong, Y.; Liu, H.; Niu, L.; Guo, J.; Liao, M.; Xiao, S.-Y. Pathological study of the 2019 novel coronavirus disease (COVID-19) through postmortem core biopsies. *Mod. Pathol.* **2020**, *33*, 1007–1014. [CrossRef]
11. Malik, P.; Patel, K.; Akrmah, M.; Donthi, D.; Patel, U.; Khader, S.N.; Asiry, S. COVID-19: A Disease with a Potpourri of Histopathologic Findings-a Literature Review and Comparison to the Closely Related SARS and MERS. *SN Compr. Clin. Med.* **2021**, *3*, 2407–2434. [CrossRef]
12. Bradley, B.T.; Maioli, H.; Johnston, R.; Chaudhry, I.; Fink, S.L.; Xu, H.; Najafian, B.; Deutsch, G.; Lacy, J.M.; Williams, T.; et al. Histopathology and ultrastructural findings of fatal COVID-19 infections in Washington State: A case series. *Lancet* **2020**, *396*, 320–332. [CrossRef]
13. Varga, Z.; Flammer, A.J.; Steiger, P.; Haberecker, M.; Andermatt, R.; Zinkernagel, A.S.; Mehra, M.R.; Schuepbach, R.A.; Ruschitzka, F.; Moch, H. Endothelial cell infection and endotheliitis in COVID-19. *Lancet* **2020**, *395*, 1417–1418. [CrossRef]
14. Wang, Y.; Liu, S.; Liu, H.; Li, W.; Lin, F.; Jiang, L.; Li, X.; Xu, P.; Zhang, L.; Zhao, L.; et al. SARS-CoV-2 infection of the liver directly contributes to hepatic impairment in patients with COVID-19. *J. Hepatol.* **2020**, *73*, 807–816. [CrossRef] [PubMed]
15. Kaltschmidt, B.; Fitzek, A.D.E.; Schaedler, J.; Förster, C.; Kaltschmidt, C.; Hansen, T.; Steinfurth, F.; Windmöller, B.A.; Pilger, C.; Kong, C.; et al. Hepatic Vasculopathy and Regenerative Responses of the Liver in Fatal Cases of COVID-19. *Clin. Gastroenterol. Hepatol.* **2021**, *19*, 1726–1729.e3. [CrossRef] [PubMed]
16. Cheung, C.C.L.; Goh, D.; Lim, X.; Tien, T.Z.; Lim, J.C.T.; Lee, J.N.; Tan, B.; Tay, Z.E.A.; Wan, W.Y.; Chen, E.X.; et al. Residual SARS-CoV-2 viral antigens detected in GI and hepatic tissues from five recovered patients with COVID-19. *Gut* **2022**, *71*, 226–229. [CrossRef] [PubMed]
17. Balaphas, A.; Gkoufa, K.; Meyer, J.; Peloso, A.; Bornand, A.; McKee, T.A.; Toso, C.; Popeskou, S.-G. COVID-19 can mimic acute cholecystitis and is associated with the presence of viral RNA in the gallbladder wall. *J. Hepatol.* **2020**, *73*, 1566–1568. [CrossRef]
18. Delorey, T.M.; Ziegler, C.G.K.; Heimberg, G.; Normand, R.; Yang, Y.; Segerstolpe, Å.; Abbondanza, D.; Fleming, S.J.; Subramanian, A.; Montoro, D.T.; et al. COVID-19 tissue atlases reveal SARS-CoV-2 pathology and cellular targets. *Nature* **2021**, *595*, 107–113. [CrossRef]
19. Pedersen, S.F.; Ho, Y.-C. SARS-CoV-2: A storm is raging. *J. Clin. Investig.* **2020**, *130*, 2202–2205. [CrossRef]
20. Pirola, C.J.; Sookoian, S. SARS-CoV-2 virus and liver expression of host receptors: Putative mechanisms of liver involvement in COVID-19. *Liver Int.* **2020**, *40*, 2038–2040. [CrossRef]
21. Senapati, S.; Banerjee, P.; Bhagavatula, S.; Kushwaha, P.P.; Kumar, S. Contributions of human ACE2 and TMPRSS2 in determining host-pathogen interaction of COVID-19. *J. Genet.* **2021**, *100*, 12. [CrossRef]
22. Jackson, C.B.; Farzan, M.; Chen, B.; Choe, H. Mechanisms of SARS-CoV-2 entry into cells. *Nat. Rev. Mol. Cell Biol.* **2022**, *23*, 3–20. [CrossRef]
23. Spearman, C.W.; Aghemo, A.; Valenti, L.; Sonderup, M.W. COVID-19 and the liver: A 2021 update. *Liver Int.* **2021**, *41*, 1988–1998. [CrossRef]
24. Yan, B.; Freiwald, T.; Chauss, D.; Wang, L.; West, E.; Mirabelli, C.; Zhang, C.J.; Nichols, E.-M.; Malik, N.; Gregory, R.; et al. SARS-CoV-2 drives JAK1/2-dependent local complement hyperactivation. *Sci. Immunol.* **2021**, *6*, eabg0833. [CrossRef]
25. Effenberger, M.; Grander, C.; Grabherr, F.; Griesmacher, A.; Ploner, T.; Hartig, F.; Bellmann-Weiler, R.; Joannidis, M.; Zoller, H.; Weiss, G.; et al. Systemic inflammation as fuel for acute liver injury in COVID-19. *Dig. Liver Dis.* **2021**, *53*, 158–165. [CrossRef]
26. Merad, M.; Blish, C.A.; Sallusto, F.; Iwasaki, A. The immunology and immunopathology of COVID-19. *Science* **2022**, *375*, 1122–1127. [CrossRef]
27. Ekpanyapong, S.; Bunchorntavakul, C.; Reddy, K.R. COVID-19 and the Liver: Lessons Learnt from the EAST and the WEST, A Year Later. *J. Viral Hepat.* **2022**, *29*, 4–20. [CrossRef]
28. Li, Y.; Xiao, S. Hepatic involvement in COVID-19 patients: Pathology, pathogenesis, and clinical implications. *J. Med. Virol.* **2020**, *92*, 1491–1494. [CrossRef]
29. Amin, M. COVID-19 and the liver: Overview. *Eur. J. Gastroenterol. Hepatol.* **2021**, *33*, 309–311. [CrossRef]
30. Eastin, C.; Eastin, T. Clinical Characteristics of Coronavirus Disease 2019 in China. *J. Emerg. Med.* **2020**, *58*, 711–712. [CrossRef]
31. Huang, C.; Wang, Y.; Li, X.; Ren, L.; Zhao, J.; Hu, Y.; Zhang, L.; Fan, G.; Xu, J.; Gu, X.; et al. Clinical features of patients infected with 2019 novel coronavirus in Wuhan, China. *Lancet* **2020**, *395*, 497–506. [CrossRef]
32. Wu, Z.; McGoogan, J.M. Characteristics of and Important Lessons From the Coronavirus Disease 2019 (COVID-19) Outbreak in China: Summary of a Report of 72 314 Cases From the Chinese Center for Disease Control and Prevention. *JAMA* **2020**, *323*, 1239–1242. [CrossRef]
33. Huang, J.; Cheng, A.; Kumar, R.; Fang, Y.; Chen, G.; Zhu, Y.; Lin, S. Hypoalbuminemia predicts the outcome of COVID-19 independent of age and co-morbidity. *J. Med. Virol.* **2020**, *92*, 2152–2158. [CrossRef]
34. Xu, Y.; Yang, H.; Wang, J.; Li, X.; Xue, C.; Niu, C.; Liao, P. Serum Albumin Levels are a Predictor of COVID-19 Patient Prognosis: Evidence from a Single Cohort in Chongqing, China. *Int. J. Gen. Med.* **2021**, *14*, 2785–2797. [CrossRef] [PubMed]

35. Ambade, V. Biochemical rationale for hypoalbuminemia in COVID-19 patients. *J. Med. Virol.* **2021**, *93*, 1207–1209. [CrossRef] [PubMed]
36. Johnson, A.; Fatemi, R.; Winlow, W. SARS-CoV-2 Bound Human Serum Albumin and Systemic Septic Shock. *Front. Cardiovasc. Med.* **2020**, *7*, 153. [CrossRef] [PubMed]
37. Liu, J.; Yu, C.; Yang, Q.; Yuan, X.; Yang, F.; Li, P.; Chen, G.; Liang, W.; Yang, Y. The clinical implication of gamma-glutamyl transpeptidase in COVID-19. *Liver Res.* **2021**, *5*, 209–216. [CrossRef]
38. Shao, T.; Tong, Y.; Lu, S.; Jeyarajan, A.J.; Su, F.; Dai, J.; Shi, J.; Huang, J.; Hu, C.; Wu, L.; et al. Gamma-Glutamyltransferase Elevation Is Frequent in Patients With COVID-19: A Clinical Epidemiologic Study. *Hepatol. Commun.* **2020**, *4*, 1744–1750. [CrossRef]
39. Zhu, X.; Wang, J.; Du, J.; Chen, S.; Chen, S.; Li, J.; Shen, B. Changes in Serum Liver Function for Patients with COVID-19: A 1-Year Follow-Up Study. *Infect. Drug Resist.* **2022**, *15*, 1857–1870. [CrossRef]
40. Sharma, A.; Nagalli, S. *Chronic Liver Disease*; StatPearls Publishing: Treasure Island, FL, USA, 2022.
41. Martinez, M.A.; Franco, S. Impact of COVID-19 in Liver Disease Progression. *Hepatol. Commun.* **2021**, *5*, 1138–1150. [CrossRef]
42. Marjot, T.; Webb, G.J.; Barritt, A.S.; Moon, A.M.; Stamataki, Z.; Wong, V.W.; Barnes, E. COVID-19 and liver disease: Mechanistic and clinical perspectives. *Nat. Rev. Gastroenterol. Hepatol.* **2021**, *18*, 348–364. [CrossRef]
43. Portincasa, P.; Krawczyk, M.; Machill, A.; Lammert, F.; Di Ciaula, A. Hepatic consequences of COVID-19 infection. Lapping or biting? *Eur. J. Intern. Med.* **2020**, *77*, 18–24. [CrossRef]
44. Marjot, T.; Moon, A.M.; Cook, J.A.; Abd-Elsalam, S.; Aloman, C.; Armstrong, M.J.; Pose, E.; Brenner, E.J.; Cargill, T.; Catana, M.-A.; et al. Outcomes following SARS-CoV-2 infection in patients with chronic liver disease: An international registry study. *J. Hepatol.* **2021**, *74*, 567–577. [CrossRef]
45. Moon, A.M.; Webb, G.J.; Aloman, C.; Armstrong, M.J.; Cargill, T.; Dhanasekaran, R.; Genescà, J.; Gill, U.S.; James, T.W.; Jones, P.D.; et al. High mortality rates for SARS-CoV-2 infection in patients with pre-existing chronic liver disease and cirrhosis: Preliminary results from an international registry. *J. Hepatol.* **2020**, *73*, 705–708. [CrossRef] [PubMed]
46. Sarin, S.K.; Choudhury, A.; Lau, G.K.; Zheng, M.-H.; Ji, D.; Abd-Elsalam, S.; Hwang, J.; Qi, X.; Cua, I.H.; Suh, J.I.; et al. APASL COVID Task Force, APASL COVID Liver Injury Spectrum Study (APCOLIS Study-NCT 04345640). Pre-existing liver disease is associated with poor outcome in patients with SARS CoV2 infection; The APCOLIS Study (APASL COVID-19 Liver Injury Spectrum Study). *Hepatol. Int.* **2020**, *14*, 690–700. [CrossRef] [PubMed]
47. Bajaj, J.S.; Garcia-Tsao, G.; Biggins, S.W.; Kamath, P.S.; Wong, F.; McGeorge, S.; Shaw, J.; Pearson, M.; Chew, M.; Fagan, A.; et al. Comparison of mortality risk in patients with cirrhosis and COVID-19 compared with patients with cirrhosis alone and COVID-19 alone: Multicentre matched cohort. *Gut* **2021**, *70*, 531–536. [CrossRef] [PubMed]
48. Iavarone, M.; D'Ambrosio, R.; Soria, A.; Triolo, M.; Pugliese, N.; Del Poggio, P.; Perricone, G.; Massironi, S.; Spinetti, A.; Buscarini, E.; et al. High rates of 30-day mortality in patients with cirrhosis and COVID-19. *J. Hepatol.* **2020**, *73*, 1063–1071. [CrossRef]
49. Kim, D.; Adeniji, N.; Latt, N.; Kumar, S.; Bloom, P.P.; Aby, E.S.; Perumalswami, P.; Roytman, M.; Li, M.; Vogel, A.S.; et al. Predictors of Outcomes of COVID-19 in Patients With Chronic Liver Disease: US Multi-center Study. *Clin. Gastroenterol. Hepatol.* **2021**, *19*, 1469–1479.e19. [CrossRef]
50. Mallet, V.; Beeker, N.; Bouam, S.; Sogni, P.; Pol, S. Demosthenes research group Prognosis of French COVID-19 patients with chronic liver disease: A national retrospective cohort study for 2020. *J. Hepatol.* **2021**, *75*, 848–855. [CrossRef]
51. Simon, T.G.; Hagström, H.; Sharma, R.; Söderling, J.; Roelstraete, B.; Larsson, E.; Ludvigsson, J.F. Risk of severe COVID-19 and mortality in patients with established chronic liver disease: A nationwide matched cohort study. *BMC Gastroenterol.* **2021**, *21*, 439. [CrossRef]
52. Nagarajan, R.; Krishnamoorthy, Y.; Rajaa, S.; Hariharan, V.S. COVID-19 Severity and Mortality Among Chronic Liver Disease Patients: A Systematic Review and Meta-Analysis. *Prev. Chronic Dis.* **2022**, *19*, E53. [CrossRef]
53. Mendizabal, M.; Ridruejo, E.; Piñero, F.; Anders, M.; Padilla, M.; Toro, L.G.; Torre, A.; Montes, P.; Urzúa, A.; Gonzalez Ballerga, E.; et al. Comparison of different prognostic scores for patients with cirrhosis hospitalized with SARS-CoV-2 infection. *Ann. Hepatol.* **2021**, *25*, 100350. [CrossRef]
54. Sharma, S.; Elhence, A.; Vaishnav, M.; Kumar, R.; Shalimar. COVID-19 in patients with cirrhosis: Understanding adverse impact. *Gut* **2021**, *70*, 1409. [CrossRef]
55. Shalimar; Elhence, A.; Vaishnav, M.; Kumar, R.; Pathak, P.; Soni, K.D.; Aggarwal, R.; Soneja, M.; Jorwal, P.; Kumar, A.; et al. Poor outcomes in patients with cirrhosis and Corona Virus Disease-19. *Indian J. Gastroenterol.* **2020**, *39*, 285–291. [CrossRef] [PubMed]
56. Warner, F.J.; Rajapaksha, H.; Shackel, N.; Herath, C.B. ACE2: From protection of liver disease to propagation of COVID-19. *Clin. Sci.* **2020**, *134*, 3137–3158. [CrossRef] [PubMed]
57. Chai, X.; Hu, L.; Zhang, Y.; Han, W.; Lu, Z.; Ke, A.; Zhou, J.; Shi, G.; Fang, N.; Fan, J.; et al. Specific ACE2 Expression in Cholangiocytes May Cause Liver Damage After 2019-nCoV Infection. *bioRxiv* **2020**. [CrossRef]
58. Gao, F.; Zheng, K.I.; Fan, Y.-C.; Targher, G.; Byrne, C.D.; Zheng, M.-H. ACE2: A Linkage for the Interplay Between COVID-19 and Decompensated Cirrhosis. *Am. J. Gastroenterol.* **2020**, *115*, 1544. [CrossRef] [PubMed]
59. Li, D.; Ding, X.; Xie, M.; Tian, D.; Xia, L. COVID-19-associated liver injury: From bedside to bench. *J. Gastroenterol.* **2021**, *56*, 218–230. [CrossRef]
60. Su, F. COVID-19 and Cirrhosis: A Combination We Must Strive to Prevent. *Gastroenterology* **2021**, *161*, 1371–1373. [CrossRef]

61. Dufour, J.-F.; Marjot, T.; Becchetti, C.; Tilg, H. COVID-19 and liver disease. *Gut* **2022**, *71*, 2350–2362. [CrossRef]
62. Ruemmele, P.; Hofstaedter, F.; Gelbmann, C.M. Secondary sclerosing cholangitis. *Nat. Rev. Gastroenterol. Hepatol.* **2009**, *6*, 287–295. [CrossRef]
63. Bütikofer, S.; Lenggenhager, D.; Wendel Garcia, P.D.; Maggio, E.M.; Haberecker, M.; Reiner, C.S.; Brüllmann, G.; Buehler, P.K.; Gubler, C.; Müllhaupt, B.; et al. Secondary sclerosing cholangitis as cause of persistent jaundice in patients with severe COVID-19. *Liver Int.* **2021**, *41*, 2404–2417. [CrossRef]
64. Ghafoor, S.; Germann, M.; Jüngst, C.; Müllhaupt, B.; Reiner, C.S.; Stocker, D. Imaging features of COVID-19-associated secondary sclerosing cholangitis on magnetic resonance cholangiopancreatography: A retrospective analysis. *Insights Imaging* **2022**, *13*, 128. [CrossRef]
65. Leonhardt, S.; Veltzke-Schlieker, W.; Adler, A.; Schott, E.; Hetzer, R.; Schaffartzik, W.; Tryba, M.; Neuhaus, P.; Seehofer, D. Trigger mechanisms of secondary sclerosing cholangitis in critically ill patients. *Crit. Care* **2015**, *19*, 131. [CrossRef] [PubMed]
66. Hunyady, P.; Streller, L.; Rüther, D.F.; Groba, S.R.; Bettinger, D.; Fitting, D.; Hamesch, K.; Marquardt, J.U.; Mücke, V.T.; Finkelmeier, F.; et al. Secondary sclerosing cholangitis following COVID-19 disease: A multicenter retrospective study. *Clin. Infect. Dis.* **2022**, ciac565. [CrossRef] [PubMed]
67. Wanner, N.; Andrieux, G.; Badia-I-Mompel, P.; Edler, C.; Pfefferle, S.; Lindenmeyer, M.T.; Schmidt-Lauber, C.; Czogalla, J.; Wong, M.N.; Okabayashi, Y.; et al. Molecular consequences of SARS-CoV-2 liver tropism. *Nat. Metab.* **2022**, *4*, 310–319. [CrossRef] [PubMed]
68. Puelles, V.G.; Lütgehetmann, M.; Lindenmeyer, M.T.; Sperhake, J.P.; Wong, M.N.; Allweiss, L.; Chilla, S.; Heinemann, A.; Wanner, N.; Liu, S.; et al. Multiorgan and Renal Tropism of SARS-CoV-2. *N. Engl. J. Med.* **2020**, *383*, 590–592. [CrossRef] [PubMed]
69. Zhao, B.; Ni, C.; Gao, R.; Wang, Y.; Yang, L.; Wei, J.; Lv, T.; Liang, J.; Zhang, Q.; Xu, W.; et al. Recapitulation of SARS-CoV-2 infection and cholangiocyte damage with human liver ductal organoids. *Protein Cell* **2020**, *11*, 771–775. [CrossRef]
70. Xu, Z.; Shi, L.; Wang, Y.; Zhang, J.; Huang, L.; Zhang, C.; Liu, S.; Zhao, P.; Liu, H.; Zhu, L.; et al. Pathological findings of COVID-19 associated with acute respiratory distress syndrome. *Lancet Respir. Med.* **2020**, *8*, 420–422. [CrossRef]
71. Tafreshi, S.; Whiteside, I.; Levine, I.; D'Agostino, C. A case of secondary sclerosing cholangitis due to COVID-19. *Clin. Imaging* **2021**, *80*, 239–242. [CrossRef]
72. Hartl, L.; Haslinger, K.; Angerer, M.; Semmler, G.; Schneeweiss-Gleixner, M.; Jachs, M.; Simbrunner, B.; Bauer, D.J.M.; Eigenbauer, E.; Strassl, R.; et al. Progressive cholestasis and associated sclerosing cholangitis are frequent complications of COVID-19 in patients with chronic liver disease. *Hepatology* **2022**, *76*, 1563–1575. [CrossRef]
73. Lee, A.; Wein, A.N.; Doyle, M.B.M.; Chapman, W.C. Liver transplantation for post-COVID-19 sclerosing cholangitis. *BMJ Case Rep.* **2021**, *14*, e244168. [CrossRef]
74. Roth, N.C.; Kim, A.; Vitkovski, T.; Xia, J.; Ramirez, G.; Bernstein, D.; Crawford, J.M. Post-COVID-19 Cholangiopathy: A Novel Entity. *Am. J. Gastroenterol.* **2021**, *116*, 1077–1082. [CrossRef]
75. Kobeszko, M.; Kumar, N. S1655 COVID-19-Induced Persistent Jaundice With Secondary Sclerosing Cholangitis. *Off. J. Am. Coll. Gastroenterol. ACG* **2021**, *116*, S741. [CrossRef]
76. Bauer, U.; Pavlova, D.; Abbassi, R.; Lahmer, T.; Geisler, F.; Schmid, R.M.; Ehmer, U. Secondary sclerosing cholangitis after COVID-19 pneumonia: A report of two cases and review of the literature. *Clin. J. Gastroenterol.* **2022**, *15*, 1124–1129. [CrossRef] [PubMed]
77. Machado, M.C.C.; Filho, R.K.; el Bacha, I.A.H.; de Oliveira, I.S.; Ribeiro, C.M.D.F.; de Souza, H.P.; Parise, E.R. Post-COVID-19 Secondary Sclerosing Cholangitis: A Rare but Severe Condition with no Treatment Besides Liver Transplantation. *Am. J. Case Rep.* **2022**, *23*, e936250. [CrossRef]
78. Browning, J.D.; Kumar, K.S.; Saboorian, M.H.; Thiele, D.L. Ethnic differences in the prevalence of cryptogenic cirrhosis. *Am. J. Gastroenterol.* **2004**, *99*, 292–298. [CrossRef] [PubMed]
79. Machado, M.V.; Diehl, A.M. Pathogenesis of Nonalcoholic Steatohepatitis. *Gastroenterology* **2016**, *150*, 1769–1777. [CrossRef]
80. Maurice, J.; Manousou, P. Non-alcoholic fatty liver disease. *Clin. Med.* **2018**, *18*, 245–250. [CrossRef]
81. Singh, A.; Hussain, S.; Antony, B. Non-alcoholic fatty liver disease and clinical outcomes in patients with COVID-19: A comprehensive systematic review and meta-analysis. *Diabetes Metab. Syndr.* **2021**, *15*, 813–822. [CrossRef]
82. Sachdeva, S.; Khandait, H.; Kopel, J.; Aloysius, M.M.; Desai, R.; Goyal, H. NAFLD and COVID-19: A Pooled Analysis. *SN Compr. Clin. Med.* **2020**, *2*, 2726–2729. [CrossRef]
83. Forlano, R.; Mullish, B.H.; Mukherjee, S.K.; Nathwani, R.; Harlow, C.; Crook, P.; Judge, R.; Soubieres, A.; Middleton, P.; Daunt, A.; et al. In-hospital mortality is associated with inflammatory response in NAFLD patients admitted for COVID-19. *PloS ONE* **2020**, *15*, e0240400. [CrossRef]
84. Younossi, Z.; Stepanova, M.; Lam, B.; Cable, R.; Felix, S.; Jeffers, T.; Younossi, E.; Pham, H.; Srishord, M.; Austin, P.; et al. Independent Predictors of Mortality Among Patients with Non-alcoholic Fatty Liver Disease (NAFLD) Hospitalized with COVID-19 Infection. *Hepatol. Commun.* **2021**, *6*, 3062–3072. [CrossRef]
85. Mushtaq, K.; Khan, M.U.; Iqbal, F.; Alsoub, D.H.; Chaudhry, H.S.; Ata, F.; Iqbal, P.; Elfert, K.; Balaraju, G.; Almaslamani, M.; et al. NAFLD is a predictor of liver injury in COVID-19 hospitalized patients but not of mortality, disease severity on the presentation or progression—The debate continues. *J. Hepatol.* **2021**, *74*, 482–484. [CrossRef] [PubMed]

86. Mahamid, M.; Nseir, W.; Khoury, T.; Mahamid, B.; Nubania, A.; Sub-Laban, K.; Schifter, J.; Mari, A.; Sbeit, W.; Goldin, E. Nonalcoholic fatty liver disease is associated with COVID-19 severity independently of metabolic syndrome: A retrospective case-control study. *Eur. J. Gastroenterol. Hepatol.* **2021**, *33*, 1578–1581. [CrossRef] [PubMed]
87. Bramante, C.T.; Tignanelli, C.J.; Dutta, N.; Jones, E.; Tamaritz, L.; Clark, J.; Melton-Meaux, G.; Usher, M.; Ikramuddin, S. Non-alcoholic fatty liver disease (NAFLD) and risk of hospitalization for Covid-19. *medRxiv* **2020**. [CrossRef]
88. Prins, G.H.; Olinga, P. Potential implications of COVID-19 in non-alcoholic fatty liver disease. *Liver Int.* **2020**, *40*, 2568. [CrossRef] [PubMed]
89. Finelli, C. Gut Microbiota, NAFLD and COVID-19: A Possible Interaction. *Obesities* **2022**, *2*, 215–221. [CrossRef]
90. Adenote, A.; Dumic, I.; Madrid, C.; Barusya, C.; Nordstrom, C.W.; Rueda Prada, L. NAFLD and Infection, a Nuanced Relationship. *Can. J. Gastroenterol. Hepatol.* **2021**, *2021*, 5556354. [CrossRef]
91. López-González, Á.A.; Altisench Jané, B.; Masmiquel Comas, L.; Arroyo Bote, S.; González San Miguel, H.M.; Ramírez Manent, J.I. Impact of COVID-19 Lockdown on Non-Alcoholic Fatty Liver Disease and Insulin Resistance in Adults: A before and after Pandemic Lockdown Longitudinal Study. *Nutrients* **2022**, *14*, 2795. [CrossRef]
92. Chang, Y.; Jeon, J.; Song, T.-J.; Kim, J. Association between the fatty liver index and the risk of severe complications in COVID-19 patients: A nationwide retrospective cohort study. *BMC Infect. Dis.* **2022**, *22*, 384. [CrossRef]
93. Ji, D.; Qin, E.; Xu, J.; Zhang, D.; Cheng, G.; Wang, Y.; Lau, G. Non-alcoholic fatty liver diseases in patients with COVID-19: A retrospective study. *J. Hepatol.* **2020**, *73*, 451–453. [CrossRef]
94. Fondevila, M.F.; Mercado-Gómez, M.; Rodríguez, A.; Gonzalez-Rellan, M.J.; Iruzubieta, P.; Valentí, V.; Escalada, J.; Schwaninger, M.; Prevot, V.; Dieguez, C.; et al. Obese patients with NASH have increased hepatic expression of SARS-CoV-2 critical entry points. *J. Hepatol.* **2021**, *74*, 469–471. [CrossRef]
95. Sharma, P.; Kumar, A.; Anikhindi, S.; Bansal, N.; Singla, V.; Shivam, K.; Arora, A. Effect of COVID-19 on Pre-existing Liver disease: What Hepatologist Should Know? *J. Clin. Exp. Hepatol.* **2021**, *11*, 484–493. [CrossRef] [PubMed]
96. Suresh Kumar, V.C.; Harne, P.S.; Mukherjee, S.; Gupta, K.; Masood, U.; Sharma, A.V.; Lamichhane, J.; Dhamoon, A.S.; Sapkota, B. Transaminitis is an indicator of mortality in patients with COVID-19: A retrospective cohort study. *World J. Hepatol.* **2020**, *12*, 619–627. [CrossRef] [PubMed]
97. Asemota, J.; Aduli, F. The Impact of Nonalcoholic Fatty Liver Disease on the Outcomes of Coronavirus Disease 2019 Infection. *Clin. Liver Dis.* **2022**, *19*, 29–31. [CrossRef] [PubMed]
98. Backer-Meurke, S.L.; Khanna, D. The Lasting Effects of COVID-19 on The Progression of Non-Alcoholic Fatty Liver Disease. *FASEB J.* **2022**, *36*. [CrossRef]
99. Milovanovic, T.; Pantic, I.; Dragasevic, S.; Lugonja, S.; Dumic, I.; Rajilic-Stojanovic, M. The interrelationship among non-alcoholic fatty liver disease, colonic diverticulosis and metabolic syndrome. *J. Gastrointestin. Liver Dis.* **2021**, *30*, 1–9. [CrossRef]
100. Wilkins, T.; Sams, R.; Carpenter, M. Hepatitis B: Screening, Prevention, Diagnosis, and Treatment. *Am. Fam. Physician* **2019**, *99*, 314–323.
101. Manns, M.P.; Maasoumy, B. Breakthroughs in hepatitis C research: From discovery to cure. *Nat. Rev. Gastroenterol. Hepatol.* **2022**, *19*, 533–550. [CrossRef]
102. Bailey, J.R.; Barnes, E.; Cox, A.L. Approaches, Progress, and Challenges to Hepatitis C Vaccine Development. *Gastroenterology* **2019**, *156*, 418–430. [CrossRef]
103. Global Hepatitis Report. 2017. Available online: https://www.who.int/publications-detail-redirect/9789241565455 (accessed on 10 September 2022).
104. Global Health Sector Strategies on, Respectively, HIV, Viral Hepatitis and Sexually Transmitted Infections for the Period 2022–2030. Available online: https://www.who.int/publications-detail-redirect/9789240053779 (accessed on 10 September 2022).
105. Yip, T.C.-F.; Gill, M.; Wong, G.L.-H.; Liu, K. Management of hepatitis B virus reactivation due to treatment of COVID-19. *Hepatol. Int.* **2022**, *16*, 257–268. [CrossRef]
106. Choe, J.W.; Jung, Y.K.; Yim, H.J.; Seo, G.H. Clinical Effect of Hepatitis B Virus on COVID-19 Infected Patients: A Nationwide Population-Based Study Using the Health Insurance Review & Assessment Service Database. *J. Korean Med. Sci.* **2022**, *37*, e29. [CrossRef]
107. Alqahtani, S.A.; Buti, M. COVID-19 and hepatitis B infection. *Antivir. Ther.* **2020**, *25*, 389–397. [CrossRef] [PubMed]
108. Wang, X.; Lei, J.; Li, Z.; Yan, L. Potential Effects of Coronaviruses on the Liver: An Update. *Front. Med.* **2021**, *8*, 651658. [CrossRef] [PubMed]
109. Yang, S.; Wang, S.; Du, M.; Liu, M.; Liu, Y.; He, Y. Patients with COVID-19 and HBV Coinfection are at Risk of Poor Prognosis. *Infect. Dis. Ther.* **2022**, *11*, 1229–1242. [CrossRef] [PubMed]
110. Chen, L.; Huang, S.; Yang, J.; Cheng, X.; Shang, Z.; Lu, H.; Cheng, J. Clinical characteristics in patients with SARS-CoV-2/HBV co-infection. *J. Viral Hepat.* **2020**, *27*, 1504–1507. [CrossRef]
111. He, Q.; Zhang, G.; Gu, Y.; Wang, J.; Tang, Q.; Jiang, Z.; Shao, C.; Zhang, H.; Chen, Z.; Ma, B.; et al. Clinical Characteristics of COVID-19 Patients With Pre-existing Hepatitis B Virus Infection: A Multicenter Report. *Am. J. Gastroenterol.* **2021**, *116*, 420–421. [CrossRef]
112. Ding, Z.-Y.; Li, G.-X.; Chen, L.; Shu, C.; Song, J.; Wang, W.; Wang, Y.-W.; Chen, Q.; Jin, G.-N.; Liu, T.-T.; et al. Association of liver abnormalities with in-hospital mortality in patients with COVID-19. *J. Hepatol.* **2021**, *74*, 1295–1302. [CrossRef]

113. Lv, X.-H.; Yang, J.-L.; Deng, K. COVID-19 Patients With Hepatitis B Virus Infection. *Am. J. Gastroenterol.* **2021**, *116*, 1357–1358. [CrossRef]
114. Kaufman, H.W.; Bull-Otterson, L.; Meyer, W.A.; Huang, X.; Doshani, M.; Thompson, W.W.; Osinubi, A.; Khan, M.A.; Harris, A.M.; Gupta, N.; et al. Decreases in Hepatitis C Testing and Treatment During the COVID-19 Pandemic. *Am. J. Prev. Med.* **2021**, *61*, 369–376. [CrossRef]
115. Mori, N.; Imamura, M.; Takaki, S.; Araki, T.; Hayes, N.C.; Aisaka, Y.; Chayama, K. Hepatitis C virus (HCV) reactivation caused by steroid therapy for dermatomyositis. *Intern. Med.* **2014**, *53*, 2689–2693. [CrossRef]
116. Lee, H.L.; Bae, S.H.; Jang, B.; Hwang, S.; Yang, H.; Nam, H.C.; Sung, P.S.; Lee, S.W.; Jang, J.W.; Choi, J.Y.; et al. Reactivation of Hepatitis C Virus and Its Clinical Outcomes in Patients Treated with Systemic Chemotherapy or Immunosuppressive Therapy. *Gut Liver* **2017**, *11*, 870–877. [CrossRef]
117. Shokri, S.; Mahmoudvand, S. The possibility of hepatitis C reactivation in COVID-19 patients treated with corticosteroids. *Ann. Hepatol.* **2022**, *27*, 100704. [CrossRef] [PubMed]
118. Afify, S.; Eysa, B.; Hamid, F.A.; Abo-Elazm, O.M.; Edris, M.A.; Maher, R.; Abdelhalim, A.; Abdel Ghaffar, M.M.; Omran, D.A.; Shousha, H.I. Survival and outcomes for co-infection of chronic hepatitis C with and without cirrhosis and COVID-19: A multicenter retrospective study. *World J. Gastroenterol.* **2021**, *27*, 7362–7375. [CrossRef] [PubMed]
119. Ronderos, D.; Omar, A.M.S.; Abbas, H.; Makker, J.; Baiomi, A.; Sun, H.; Mantri, N.; Choi, Y.; Fortuzi, K.; Shin, D.; et al. Chronic hepatitis-C infection in COVID-19 patients is associated with in-hospital mortality. *World J. Clin. Cases* **2021**, *9*, 8749–8762. [CrossRef] [PubMed]
120. Hamid, S.; Alvares da Silva, M.R.; Burak, K.W.; Chen, T.; Drenth, J.P.H.; Esmat, G.; Gaspar, R.; LaBrecque, D.; Lee, A.; Macedo, G.; et al. WGO Guidance for the Care of Patients With COVID-19 and Liver Disease. *J. Clin. Gastroenterol.* **2021**, *55*, 1–11. [CrossRef] [PubMed]
121. Elfiky, A.A. Ribavirin, Remdesivir, Sofosbuvir, Galidesivir, and Tenofovir against SARS-CoV-2 RNA dependent RNA polymerase (RdRp): A molecular docking study. *Life Sci.* **2020**, *253*, 117592. [CrossRef] [PubMed]
122. Gadour, E.; Hassan, Z.; Shrwani, K. P31 Covid-19 induced hepatitis (CIH), definition and diagnostic criteria of a poorly understood new clinical syndrome. *Gut* **2020**, *69*, A22. [CrossRef]
123. Balaja, W.R.; Jacob, S.; Hamidpour, S.; Masoud, A. COVID-19 Presenting as Acute Icteric Hepatitis. *Cureus* **2021**, *13*, e16359. [CrossRef]
124. Wang, Z.-Z.; Li, K.; Maskey, A.R.; Huang, W.; Toutov, A.A.; Yang, N.; Srivastava, K.; Geliebter, J.; Tiwari, R.; Miao, M.; et al. A small molecule compound berberine as an orally active therapeutic candidate against COVID-19 and SARS: A computational and mechanistic study. *FASEB J.* **2021**, *35*, e21360. [CrossRef]
125. Ghareeb, D.A.; Saleh, S.R.; Seadawy, M.G.; Nofal, M.S.; Abdulmalek, S.A.; Hassan, S.F.; Khedr, S.M.; AbdElwahab, M.G.; Sobhy, A.A.; Abdel-Hamid, A.S.A.; et al. Nanoparticles of ZnO/Berberine complex contract COVID-19 and respiratory co-bacterial infection in addition to elimination of hydroxychloroquine toxicity. *J. Pharm. Investig.* **2021**, *51*, 735–757. [CrossRef]
126. Warowicka, A.; Nawrot, R.; Goździcka-Józefiak, A. Antiviral activity of berberine. *Arch. Virol.* **2020**, *165*, 1935–1945. [CrossRef]
127. Hung, T.-C.; Jassey, A.; Liu, C.-H.; Lin, C.-J.; Lin, C.-C.; Wong, S.H.; Wang, J.Y.; Yen, M.-H.; Lin, L.-T. Berberine inhibits hepatitis C virus entry by targeting the viral E2 glycoprotein. *Phytomedicine* **2019**, *53*, 62–69. [CrossRef] [PubMed]
128. Kim, S.-Y.; Kim, H.; Kim, S.-W.; Lee, N.-R.; Yi, C.-M.; Heo, J.; Kim, B.-J.; Kim, N.-J.; Inn, K.-S. An Effective Antiviral Approach Targeting Hepatitis B Virus with NJK14047, a Novel and Selective Biphenyl Amide p38 Mitogen-Activated Protein Kinase Inhibitor. *Antimicrob. Agents Chemother.* **2017**, *61*, e00214-17. [CrossRef] [PubMed]
129. Jena, A.B.; Kanungo, N.; Chainy, G.B.N.; Devaraji, V.; Das, S.K.; Dandapat, J. A Computational Insight on the Inhibitory Potential of 8-Hydroxydihydrosanguinarine (8-HDS), a Pyridone Containing Analog of Sanguinarine, against SARS CoV2. *Chem. Biodivers.* **2022**, *19*, e202200266. [CrossRef] [PubMed]

Disclaimer/Publisher's Note: The statements, opinions and data contained in all publications are solely those of the individual author(s) and contributor(s) and not of MDPI and/or the editor(s). MDPI and/or the editor(s) disclaim responsibility for any injury to people or property resulting from any ideas, methods, instructions or products referred to in the content.

Review

Drug-Induced Liver Injury in Hospitalized Patients during SARS-CoV-2 Infection

Eleni Karlafti [1,2,*], Daniel Paramythiotis [3], Konstantina Pantazi [2], Vasiliki Epameinondas Georgakopoulou [4], Georgia Kaiafa [2], Petros Papalexis [5,6], Adonis A. Protopapas [2], Eleftheria Ztriva [2], Varvara Fyntanidou [1] and Christos Savopoulos [2]

1. Emergency Department, AHEPA University General Hospital, Aristotle University of Thessaloniki, 54636 Thessaloniki, Greece
2. First Propaedeutic Department of Internal Medicine, AHEPA University General Hospital, Aristotle University of Thessaloniki, 54636 Thessaloniki, Greece
3. First Propaedeutic Department of Surgery, AHEPA University General Hospital, Aristotle University of Thessaloniki, 54636 Thessaloniki, Greece
4. Pulmonology Department, Laiko General Hospital, Medical School, National and Kapodistrian University of Athens, 11527 Athens, Greece
5. Unit of Endocrinology, First Department of Internal Medicine, Laiko General Hospital, National and Kapodistrian University of Athens, 11527 Athens, Greece
6. Department of Biomedical Sciences, University of West Attica, 12243 Athens, Greece
* Correspondence: linakarlafti@hotmail.com; Tel.: +231-330-3110

Abstract: In the last few years, the world has had to face the SARS-CoV-2 infection and its multiple effects. Even though COVID-19 was first considered to be a respiratory disease, it has an extended clinical spectrum with symptoms occurring in many tissues, and it is now identified as a systematic disease. Therefore, various drugs are used during the therapy of hospitalized COVID-19 patients. Studies have shown that many of these drugs could have adverse side-effects, including drug-induced liver injury—also known as DILI—which is the focus of our review. Despite the consistent findings, the pathophysiological mechanism behind DILI in COVID-19 disease is still complex, and there are a few risk factors related to it. However, when it comes to the diagnosis, there are specific algorithms (including the RUCAM algorithm) and biomarkers that can assist in identifying DILI and which we will analyze in our review. As indicated by the title, a variety of drugs are associated with this COVID-19-related complication, including systemic corticosteroids, drugs used for the therapy of uncontrolled cytokine storm, as well as antiviral, anti-inflammatory, and anticoagulant drugs. Bearing in mind that hepatotoxicity is very likely to occur during COVID-19, especially in patients treated with multiple medications, we will also refer to the use of other drugs used for DILI therapy in an effort to control and prevent a severe and long-term outcome.

Keywords: drug-induced liver injury (DILI); COVID-19; liver injury; liver dysfunction; COVID-19 treatment; liver function; COVID-19 drugs

1. Introduction

Since 2019, the world has had to face the virus SARS-CoV-2 and its multiple effects. Currently, COVID-19 is considered to be a systemic disease, with a large variety of symptoms noted among patients. Many patients even end up being hospitalized for the detrimental health problems it causes. Multiple drugs are used as medications for COVID-19 and its symptoms, which are more commonly located in the respiratory system and include—but are not restricted to—fever, cough, shortness of breath, and pneumonia [1]. However, COVID-19 symptoms are not only located in the respiratory system [2]. They can reach several systems through the angiotensin-converting enzyme receptor 2 (ACE-2), which is present in numerous tissues, such as the gastrointestinal tract, the vascular endothelium, and the liver. Therefore, the viral infection can reach all the tissues where the ACE-2 receptor is located [1].

Specifically regarding the liver, studies have shown that the ACE-2 receptor is expressed in the liver tissue and expressly, in the hepatocytes (2.9%), but even more intensely in the cholangiocytes (59.7%) [3]. Interestingly, it has been proven that ACE-2 expression in the cholangiocytes is similar to that in type 2 pneumonocytes [4]. In other words, the liver is a target organ for COVID-19. The frequency of liver damage ranges from 14.8% to 53% among COVID-19 patients [5]. Liver disease during COVID-19 can be attributed to many factors (Figure 1), such as virus-related cytopathic injury [1], direct hepatocellular damage through the ACE-2 receptor [6,7], (Figure 1), uncontrolled inflammatory reaction leading to fibrosis and liver dysfunction, septic shock [1], hypoxia [8] and reoxygenation [1], cholestatic damage, or even thrombosis due to the hypercoagulable state created by the virus' effect on the vascular endothelium [1].

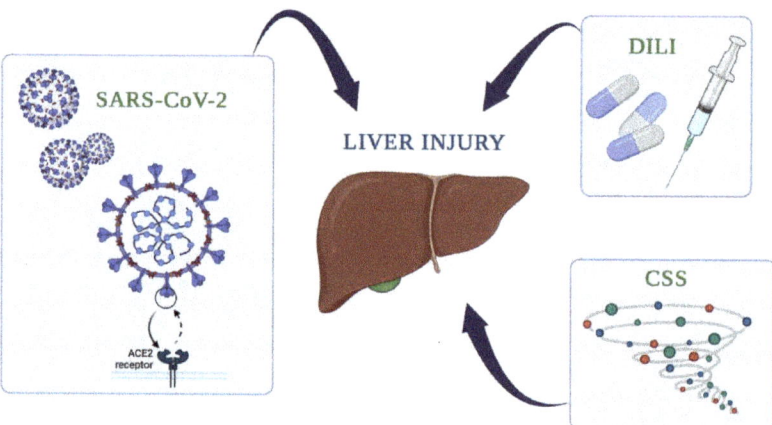

Figure 1. Liver injury during COVID-19 infection can occur through multiple pathways. A few common examples are pictured above, and they include: direct injury through the ACE-2 receptor, uncontrolled general inflammation as a result of the cytokine storm syndrome (CSS), and drug-induced liver injury (DILI).

Liver injury is also common as a result of drug administration (Figure 1). At the beginning of the pandemic, there was no definitive treatment for COVID-19; however, currently, there are several possible medications. Especially at first, many caregivers proposed the use of antiviral drugs and monoclonal antibodies, antibiotics, immunomodulator agents, non-steroidal anti-inflammatory drugs, steroids, antipyretic medicine, and complementary treatments [7,8]. However, these drugs, like most medications, can have side effects, with hepatotoxicity being a common result. It is important to mention that the occurrence and the level of liver damage depend on many factors, such as the medicine dose and patient characteristics. It is also interesting to mention that there are some intrinsic liver diseases that predispose the development of DILI, with a common condition being non-alcoholic fatty liver disease (NAFLD) [9]. As a matter of fact, the risk of DILI during COVID-19 infection is higher in patients with NAFLD [10]. NAFLD makes hepatocytes more fragile during COVID-19 infection and more vulnerable to medications, especially antipyretic drugs containing acetaminophen [7].

In this review, our goal is to explain the association between liver injury in COVID-19 patients and the medications used as therapeutic strategies for COVID-19 treatment. Drug-induced liver injury (DILI) is a common cause of hepatotoxicity and hepatic damage during COVID-19.

2. Materials and Methods

Before synthesizing this review, comprehensive research on drug-induced liver damage caused by COVID-19 medications was performed. All the research was conducted up until August 2022, with the main database used being PubMed. All the sources were in the English language. Multiple reviews and articles were thoroughly studied in order to synthesize a holistic review of DILI during COVID-19 infection.

Since the goal of this review is to exhibit a complete depiction of DILI during COVID-19 infection and bearing in mind that the COVID-19 pandemic is still active, no limitations were set regarding the number of sources or the date of their release. Moreover, since the COVID-19 pandemic afflicted most countries, no geographical limitations were set. It is also important to mention that our goal was to not only to refer to common COVID-19 medications, but also to mention most of the drugs that have been considered as COVID-19 therapies.

Additionally, part of our research also focused on the tests executed in order to diagnose the DILI, as well as on the risk factors that could possibly add to the possibility of DILI. Moreover, we also decided to investigate DILI prophylaxis and possible therapeutic strategies for the occurrence of liver damage.

The main keywords and key phrases used as a basis for our research were "COVID-19," "SARS-CoV-2," "drug-induced liver injury," "DILI," "liver injury," "liver dysfunction," "COVID-19 treatment," "liver function," and "COVID-19 drugs."

3. Discussion

3.1. All about DILI

3.1.1. General Information

DILI is a liver injury caused by medication [7]. Even though DILI is not common, it is a frequent cause of liver dysfunction and acute liver failure in hospitalized patients [4]. It frequently occurs in hospitalized COVID-19 patients, especially when they are treated with multiple drug regimens, which is quite common [4].

DILI can be hepatocellular, cholestatic, or mixed, the most common type being hepatocellular. DILI is characterized as hepatocellular when a five-fold or higher rise in ALT alone is noted, or when the ratio of serum ALP to ALT is five or more times the ULN [11]. On the other hand, when there a two-fold or higher rise in ALP alone, or when the ratio of serum ALP to ALT is two or less times the ULN, the DILI is termed as cholestatic [11]. The condition where the ratio of serum ALT to ALP is higher than two times and lower than five times the ULN is called mixed DILI [11].

From a different approach, DILI can be either intrinsic or idiosyncratic. Intrinsic DILI is infrequent. However, it is predictable, dose dependent, and it occurs after a short latency period [6]. The most common drug that induces intrinsic DILI is paracetamol or acetaminophen [6]. In contrast, idiosyncratic DILI is the most common type of DILI, but it is unpredictable, with a latency period that can last up to a few months [6].

It is also interesting to mention that DILI patterns differ between the different types of causative medications. For instance, studies have shown an association between cephalosporins and hepatobiliary adverse drug reactions (ADRs) [12]. At the same time, drugs such as ciprofloxacin can lead to idiosyncratic DILI (even though it is rare) because ciprofloxacin is infrequently associated with liver toxicity [13]. The medications that most often cause DILI are antimicrobials [13].

As for the progression of DILI, it varies from mild to severe, with extreme cases leading to liver transplant [6,14]. Under all circumstances, pre-existing chronic liver disease will result in a worse prognosis and a mortality rate three times higher than that in patients with a healthy liver [6]. Sources also state that patients with liver steatosis and metabolic syndrome are more prone to contract DILI after COVID-19 [15].

3.1.2. Mechanism of DILI

Even though the mechanisms that lead to DILI are not fully understood, there are multiple pathways that result in the sensitization of the hepatocytes and the induction of liver damage. Drug-induced steatosis in the liver tissues of COVID-19 patients is one of the medical conditions in which drug administration can lead to liver injury. According to Xu et al., microvesicular steatosis in the liver of COVID-19 patients is a condition where the hepatocytes are filled with fat vesicles due to viral or drug-induced liver damage [16]. Steatosis caused by medications is, in many cases, caused by drug interference with the β-oxidation of fatty acids, mitochondrial respiration, or both [7]. This reaction subsequently results in the accretion of non-esterified fatty acids, which are later converted into triglycerides [7].

Another mechanism that affects the hepatocytes and is worth mentioning is the downregulation of cytochromes p450 (CYPs) [7]. These cytochromes are enzymes involved in the oxidative biotransformation of many medications used in COVID-19 therapy [17]. The downregulation occurs because of the increase in cytokines and interleukins caused by the cytokine storm syndrome during COVID-19 [17]. Specifically, IL-6 is a significant inflammatory mediator, that exerts repressive effects on many CYPs [17]. The suppression of CYPs affects the metabolism of many COVID-19 drugs, especially remdesivir [17].

3.1.3. DILI Risk Factors

In a study done by Delgado et al. on 36,905 hospitalized patients, out of whom 8719 were diagnosed with COVID-19, 160 (1.8%) of the COVID-19 patients were also diagnosed with DILI [18]. Out of these 160 patients, 124 (77.5%) were men, and the mean age was 54.3 years [18]. This leads to the conclusion that men around the age of 50 are more prone to DILI during COVID-19 [18,19]. In addition, a review conducted by Teschke et al. concluded that the male-to-female ratio for DILI during COVID-19 was around 2.6:1 [20], which implicates that men are more vulnerable to DILI than women. Another risk factor is pregnancy, with the difference being that it affects only cholestatic or mixed liver injury and not hepatocellular injury [19]. However, there are only limited data supporting that pregnant women are more vulnerable to DILI. As a matter of fact, tetracycline seems to be the only drug known to increase the risk of DILI during pregnancy [21].

Moreover, according to the same study by Delgado et al., many of the 160 patients also exhibited multiple comorbidities [18]. Specifically, 71 (44.4%) had dyslipidemia, 49 (30.6%) had high blood pressure, and 11 (6.8%) had diabetes mellitus. Additionally, 14 (8.8%) patients were smokers, while 6 (3.8%) were systematically consuming alcohol [18]. Alcohol consumption is a common risk factor for DILI, but it is only associated with specific medications. Moreover, alcohol can trigger DILI after long-term consumption of more than two alcoholic drinks per day, for women, and more than three alcoholic drinks per day for men [19].

A risk factor that cannot be ignored is the presence of pre-existing liver injuries (e.g., fatty liver) or viral infections (e.g., hepatitis C or HIV virus) [22,23]. To make things clearer, pre-existing liver injuries and infections can be considered as risk factors due to the drugs administered as therapeutic approaches [24]. There is also a hypothesis that obese COVID-19 patients with NAFLD could potentially be at a higher risk for DILI than patients who have not been infected by SARS-CoV-2 or non-obese NAFLD patients [23]. This hypothesis is attributed to the fact that obese COVID-19 patients with NAFLD are simultaneously included in the spectrum of multiple risk factors for DILI [23].

The development of DILI also depends on the medications used. By definition, DILI is caused by drugs, so every hepatotoxic drug could induce liver damage. However, as many studies have shown, the chances of DILI are much higher when multiple drugs or higher doses are administered [25,26]. It is a fact that patients that are treated with five or more drugs, such as ICU patients, are more likely to develop DILI [1].

3.1.4. DILI Diagnosis

When it comes to the diagnosis of DILI, it is usually quite challenging, as it is a diagnosis made by elimination. When collecting the patient's history, a physician that suspects the presence of DILI should not omit questions about alcohol abuse, chronic or acute liver diseases, other comorbidities, and the medications (including herbal and dietary supplements) that the patient has consumed, especially in the last six months [6]. Additionally, laboratory tests to detect viral hepatitis or autoimmune hepatic diseases should be conducted, while imaging of the liver should be performed when there is suspicion of a preexisting liver disease or in order to exclude vascular, biliar or neoplastic disorders. Conducting an abdominal doppler ultrasound examination is also important in order to exclude the possibility of vascular liver disease, such as hepatic vein or portal vein thrombosis. Furthermore, liver biopsy should be considered in patients where an alternative diagnosis is probable, as well as in patients where DILI does not resolve, despite the withdrawal of possible causative agents.

DILI can be diagnosed by an elevation in liver enzymes, which can occur due to hepatocellular necrosis, cholestasis, or both. These laboratory changes are not always accompanied by symptoms [6]. Common and useful findings in the laboratory results of hospitalized COVID-19 patients with liver damage are elevated aspartate aminotransferase (AST) and increased alanine aminotransferase (ALT), specifically ALT >3 times ULN [1,6]. Other less-frequent findings include a decrease in serum albumin and an increase in total bilirubin >2 times the normal upper limit [1], in gamma-glutamyl transferase (GGT) and in alkaline phosphatase levels (ALP) [1,6]. One could also measure the prolonged prothrombin time (ppt), which mirrors the alteration of the hepatic synthesis of coagulation factors [23]. All these biomarkers can be measured within the plasma using liver function tests (LFTs) [23].

3.1.5. RUCAM

A widely used test that can assist in the diagnosis of DILI is the Roussel Uclaf Causality Assessment Method (RUCAM). It helps to identify both DILI and other liver diseases. It is very useful in order to assess the causality and the level of liver injury when DILI is suspected, allowing caregivers to take proper treatment measures. The RUCAM scale is a point system based on seven domains, which include the temporal evolution of the liver damage, risk factors, concomitant use of possibly hepatotoxic drugs, and the reoccurrence of liver injury after a new drug is used [1]. RUCAM was the first method to establish valid criteria for liver injury caused by hepatotoxic drugs, thus eliminating cases with nonspecific elevated liver enzymes without clinical relevance [19].

When using the RUCAM, the limits for DILI diagnosis are a serum ALT at least five times ULN and/or a serum ALP at least two times the ULN [6,19]. These criteria help specify the hepatotoxicity causality assessment and eliminate false positive tests [19]. It is important to note that when ALT levels are normal and ALP levels are elevated, further biomarkers should be examined. Specifically, there should also be an increase in γ-glutamyl transpeptidase, in order to reject cases of ALP elevation through other sources.

RUCAM can even differentiate if the liver injury is hepatocellular or cholestatic. Liver injury can be identified as hepatocellular when ALT > 5 times ULN and ALP $\leq$ 2 times ULN, or if both are elevated, R $\geq$ 5, with R = ALT/ALP. The liver injury is cholestatic when ALP > 2 times ULN and ALT $\leq$ 1-time ULN, or if both ALT and ALP are elevated, R $\leq$ 2, and mixed when ALT > 5 times ULN and ALP > 1 times ULN and 2 < R < 5 [19].

Even though RUCAM shows high sensitivity (86%) and specificity (89%), it can primarily assess DILI when studying single drug cases. When it comes to polypharmacy, RUCAM shows a poor discrimination value [18]. The limitations of RUCAM have led to the development of another assessment method, the revised electronic causality assessment method (RECAM). RECAM diagnostic categories are more compatible with expert opinion and are much more sensitive in comparison to RUCAM, especially when it comes to the detection of extreme diagnostic categories [27]. Therefore, RECAM is believed to be more precise and reliable for DILI diagnosis [27].

Another test that can be used to assess DILI under conditions of polypharmacy, is the lymphocyte transformation test (LTT), which assesses the proliferation of T cells due to in vitro drug exposure [28]. It is used to prove whether a patient has been sensitized to specific drugs [18], however, it is not standard nor general.

3.1.6. DILI Associated Medications

Many of the drugs that are administered as a treatment for COVID-19 (e.g., lopinavir/ritonavir, hydroxychloroquine) are metabolized in the liver, thus causing liver damage and elevated liver enzymes [7]. DILI during COVID-19 depends on the type of drug that causes it [7]. Cai et al. proved that drugs such as antibiotics and non-steroidal anti-inflammatory drugs (NSAIDs) are not as hepatotoxic as antiviral drugs, such as lopinavir/ritonavir, which are much more likely to cause DILI [29].

Moreover, when it comes to liver injury, some drugs (e.g., azithromycin, chloroquine) are hepatotoxic in the presence of a mild inflammation [18]. This has also been proven in animal studies [18] and can be explained by the fact that reactive drug metabolites are produced by inflammatory cells during inflammation [18]. More specifically, myeloperoxidase is an enzyme derived from inflammatory cells that can convert specific drugs to reactive cytotoxic metabolites [18].

Multiple medications can lead to hepatotoxic effects. The hepatotoxic profiles of drugs commonly administered as part of COVID-19 treatment are displayed in Figure 2. These include systemic corticosteroids; antiviral drugs such as remdesivir, lopinavir/ritonavir, and favipiravir (FRP); antibiotics such as azithromycin; antimalarials such as hydroxychloroquine; immunomodulatory agents such as tocilizumab (TCZ) and sarilumab; antipyretics, including paracetamol; NSAIDs; colchicine; low molecular weight heparins; (LMWH) and molnupiravir.

MEDICATION	TYPE	LIVER CONTRAINDICATIONS	DILI PATTERN
Systemic corticosteroids	systemic corticosteroids	caution in LF	hepatocellular / mixed
Remdesivir	antiviral drug	ALT>10 x ULN or ALT>5 x ULN + symptoms	hepatocellular
Lopinavir/Ritonavir	antiviral drug	ALT>5 x ULN	hepatocellular
Favipiravir	antiviral drug	↑FRP, ALT, AST, ALP, total bilirubin levels	cholestatic + hepatocellular
Azithromycin	antibiotic	ALT>5 x ULN + dermal reactions	hepatocellular / mixed
Hydroxychloroquine	antimalarials	ALT elevation	-
Tocilizumab	monoclonal antibody	ALT>5 x ULN	hepatocellular
Sarilumab	monoclonal antibody	ALT>1.5 x ULN	hepatocellular
Paracetamol	antipyretic	MAFLD/NAFLD, alcoholic patients	hepatocellular
NSAIDs	NSAIDs	caution in LF, contradiciton in severe LF	hepatocellular
Colchicine	anti-gout agent	dosing restrictions in liver dysfunction	-
LMWH	LMWH	caution in LF	hepatocellular

Figure 2. COVID-19 medications that can cause DILI, the category in which they belong, the liver contraindications that exist, and the DILI patterns that they develop. Abbreviations used: NSAIDs—non-steroidal anti-inflammatory drugs; LMWH—low molecular weight heparins; LF—liver failure; ALT—alanine aminotransferase; ULN—upper limit of normal; FRP—favipiravir; AST—aspartate aminotransferase; ALP—alkaline phosphatase; MAFLD—metabolic associated fatty liver disease; NAFLD—non-alcoholic fatty liver disease. The arrow used in this figure signifies elevation of the mentioned biomarkers.

3.2. Ketamine

Before focusing on the medications that lead to DILI, a special mention should be made concerning ketamine, which is not a drug, but an analgesic sedative. During COVID-19 hospitalization, many mechanically ventilated patients struggle with symptoms such as acute respiratory distress syndrome (ARDS), which require large doses of analgesic sedatives [30] for lung protective mechanical ventilation. For this purpose, drugs such as ketamine, an N-methyl-D-aspartate (NMDA) receptor antagonist with both sedative and analgesic properties, are commonly administrated in the ICU as anesthetics [31].

The long-term infusion of ketamine, however, can exhibit a dose-dependent relationship with elevated bilirubin levels and a higher risk of cholestatic liver injury in COVID-19 patients with ARDS [31]. The short-term infusion of ketamine (e.g., 72 h) is probably not likely to cause the development of its hazardous effects. An analysis executed by Wendel-Garcia et al. shows that the increase in bilirubin by 15 μmol/L and in ALP by 150 U/L is only noticeable after ketamine administration of 1.5 mg/kg/h for 14 days straight [31]. Bearing this in mind, it is suggested that the long-term infusion of high-dose ketamine in mechanically ventilated COVID-19 patients be avoided [31]. When ketamine is used, it is vital to monitor bilirubin and ALP levels daily [31].

3.3. Systemic Corticosteroids

Systemic corticosteroids are often used in COVID-19 patients, even though they tend to have multiple adverse effects, including hyperglycemia and secondary infections [6]. DILI can also occur from corticosteroids, even though the chances are very slim [6]. Some authors even suggest their use as a treatment for severe DILI [32], while other authors are hesitant regarding this recommendation [33].

Since corticosteroid-induced liver injury during SARS-CoV-2 infection is infrequent, only a few cases have been documented. A study performed in Hong Kong in a cohort of 1040 patients showed that the administration of corticosteroids was independently related to liver injury. This was attributed either to the fact that patients with COVID-19 who used corticosteroids were already severely ill and thus, more prone to factors that could affect their liver function [6], or to the fact that corticosteroids can promote non-alcoholic steatohepatitis (NASH) in patients with NAFLD [6], or even exacerbate a pre-existing steatosis [23].

3.4. Antiviral Drugs

3.4.1. Remdesivir

Antivirals are regularly used for treating COVID-19, with remdesivir being a common antiviral drug recommendation [6], since it has shown to promote higher survival rates among adult COVID-19 patients [34]. Moreover, remdesivir is highly used because it has been proven to be superior to placebo in decreasing recovery time for hospitalized patients [35]. Remdesivir is an active inhibitor of viral RNA-dependent RNA polymerases [6], with a documented hepatotoxicity potential [4]. According to a study by Delgado et al., remdesivir has the highest incidence rate of DILI per administration [18], while another study by Kaur et al. reported the first case of DILI caused by remdesivir in a newborn with COVID-19 [34].

When administering remdesivir for COVID-19, the standard dose is 200 mg the first day and then 100 mg daily for 4 to 9 days [6]. In hospitalized COVID-19 patients in need of oxygen supplementation, remdesivir's beneficial effects are notable within ten days from the beginning of the symptoms [6].

On the other hand, one common adverse effect of remdesivir on the liver of COVID-19 patients is the elevation of serum aminotransferase and ALP levels [6,18,36,37], with a range of 15–20% [38]. Other significant symptoms, such as jaundice, are absent [6]. However, the presence of pre-existing liver failure and creatine clearance below 30 mL/min are contraindications for remdesivir administration, as it causes the elevation of transaminases [34]. Remdesivir-induced liver injury is most likely based on the interaction of P-glycoprotein (P-gp) inhibitors [39]. Remdesivir-induced DILI can also occur through the decrease in its metabolism, due to CYPs' downregulation during the cytokine storm [7]. Accordingly, remdesivir should be used with caution, and reserved only for severe COVID-19 infections [34].

In order to control remdesivir's effects, LFTs should be executed before and during remdesivir use. In the case that ALT levels increase >10 times ULN, or there are symptoms accompanied by a smaller ALT elevation, remdesivir therapy should be terminated [40]. A case report by Carothers et al. suggested the use of acetylcysteine for managing acute liver failure (ALF) induced by remdesivir [41]. Acetylcysteine is an antidote to acetaminophen, which is the leading cause of ALF. However, acetylcysteine can also be used to treat ALF caused by other drugs [7].

3.4.2. Protease Inhibitors: Lopinavir/Ritonavir

In a review done by Kulkarni et al., it was shown that the incidence of lopinavir/ritonavir (LPV/r)-induced liver injury in COVID-19 patients was 37.2% among 775 COVID-19 patients [37]. In another study by Batteux et al., where 65 hospitalized COVID-19 patients were treated with LPV/r, 25 (38.5%) developed liver damage [42]. Moreover, Cai et al., after studying 417 COVID-19 patients, concluded that the risk of liver damage in patients who took LPV/R was increased four-fold compared to patients who did not follow this treatment [29].

The most common side effects of LPV/r treatment were hyperbilirubinemia and elevated liver enzymes, especially GGT [29,37,43]. The elevation of serum concentration of aminotransferases (>5 times ULN) is mainly attributed to lopinavir, while ritonavir rarely results in alterations in liver enzyme concentrations [7].

The combination of lopinavir and ritonavir overdose could lead to the activation of the endoplasmic reticulum stress pathway in the liver. When this pathway is triggered, it can subsequently induce hepatocyte apoptosis through the caspase cascade system. This can further lead to inflammation and oxidative stress and thus, accelerate liver injury. However, it is important to note that LPV/r affects liver function in a dose-dependent manner [43].

Out of these two protease inhibitors, ritonavir and full-dose ritonavir treatment seem to be associated with a higher risk of DILI [18]. Ritonavir, specifically, is a CEA4 inhibitor [18] and is metabolized by the liver with the mediation of the cytochrome P450 (cytochrome P3A4/CYP3A4) pathway [4]. Even though the cause of liver enzyme elevation after ritonavir medication is not fully known [4], the basis of the liver damage is believed to be the production of a toxic intermediate of ritonavir or other drugs metabolized by CYP3A4> [4]. For example, both Arbidol and lopinavir are metabolized by CYP3A, which ritonavir inhibits. Therefore, when using Arbidol and LPV/R simultaneously, liver injury can occur [7].

3.4.3. Favipiravir

FRP is a pyrazinecarboxamide derivative antiviral drug not believed to cause liver injury when administered alone. However, a study by Yamazaki et al. refers to a COVID-19 patient who developed cholestatic liver injury after being treated with FRP [44]. The author asserts that the liver injury was induced by the prior treatment with antibacterial therapy, which was worsened by FRP [44]. FRP's chemical structure implies that it has the potential to cause liver damage [7], due to the fact that it is structurally similar to pyrazinamide, which is typically hepatotoxic [7], but the chemical structure remains unclear [7].

In patients with FRP-induced liver injury, elevated levels of serum FRP are noted [7]. As a matter of fact, FRP levels were more elevated in patients with liver injury than in the patients who took FRP, but did not have FRP-induced liver damage. This leads to the conclusion that monitoring FRP concentration is essential in order to be able to keep track of FRP's effects on the patients' livers and regulate the ideal FRP dose [7].

3.5. Antibiotics—Azithromycin

It is rather interesting that about 75% of COVID-19 patients—hospitalized or not—are prescribed antibiotics, while the estimated bacterial infection rate is only 8.6% [6]. Several antibiotics can induce liver injury, with a relatively common one being azithromycin.

Azithromycin, a broad-spectrum macrolide, is one of the drugs that was widely used during the beginning of the COVID-19 pandemic [6], since it decreases inflammatory cytokines (ex. IL-6, IL-8, TNF-α) and reduces oxidative stress [45,46]. The main adverse effect of azithromycin use is its cardiac toxicity, especially when in combination with hydroxychloroquine, though it has also been associated with hepatotoxicity [6], especially in patients with pre-existing liver damage [6,33]. In a study conducted by Delgado et al., azithromycin exhibited the second-highest incidence rate of DILI, after remdesivir [18].

Azithromycin-induced liver damage usually occurs within 1–3 weeks after the beginning of the treatment, while the hepatocellular injury it causes has a short latency [7]. Moreover, azithromycin can also contribute to the development of dermal reactions that are associated with liver injury, such as erythema multiforme and Stevens–Johnson syndrome [7]. The liver tests from COVID-19 patients with azithromycin-induced liver injury include an ALT elevation <6 ULN in 40% of the patients [23].

3.6. Antimalarials—Hydroxychloroquine

Hydroxychloroquine (HCQ), as a COVID-19 medication, is also related to DILI [18]. In a study, Falcao et al. reported a severe case of HCQ-induced liver injury during COVID-19 hospitalization. Specifically, the patient being studied showed a 10-fold elevation in serum transaminase levels while on HCQ and a sudden decrease after quitting HCQ therapy [7]. Moreover, Rismanbaf et al. showed that the association between the inflammatory response to COVID-19 infection and an adverse reaction to the reactive metabolite of HCQ could lead to liver injury [47].

However, it is important to mention that there are also studies, such as the one done by Kelly et al., which report that adverse effects on the liver were not significantly different between patients using HCQ and azithromycin and the effects noted in the control group [48].

3.7. Immunomodulatory Therapies: Tocilizumab and Sarilumab

Severe COVID-19 infection is followed by a systemic inflammation that leads to the cytokine storm or cytokine release syndrome (CRS). This overproduction of cytokines is characterized by—among other indications—an increase in the concentrations of interleukin (IL)-6, C-reactive protein (CRP), D-dimer, and ferritin [6], which can result in rather detrimental effects, such as multi-organ damage [6]. Multiple medications are considered as treatments for this situation, with the most used being TCZ, which is an extendedly studied recombinant monoclonal antibody that fulfills the role of an IL-6R antagonist [6,49]. TCZ is usually administrated to patients with severe lung injury and elevated IL-6 blood levels [22]. It is usually combined with dexamethasone for patients with rapid respiratory decompensation [50].

Studies have shown that TCZ does indeed assist in the decrease in overactive inflammation and the need for intubation [50]. However, it has also been proven to have side effects, including immune suppression and hepatotoxicity [6], which occur through mechanisms that are not well-understood [7]. Immunosuppressants (TCZ, dexamethasone, and tofacitinib) can further increase the risk of fulminant liver failure due to the reactivation of hepatitis B virus (HBV) infection in chronic carriers [22,51]. In some cases of treatment with TCZ that led to acute liver failure and acute hepatitis, liver transplant was required [4]. HBV screening for patients who are considered to be candidates for intense immunosuppressive treatment would help eliminate cases of acute hepatitis B.

The liver injury caused by TCZ, which is dose-dependent, is mainly identified through the elevation of transaminase levels, while other side effects have yet to be noted [6]. TCZ hepatotoxic status is mainly visible when combined with other potentially hepatotoxic drugs. For instance, a study by Guaraldi et al. on 1351 patients treated with TCZ concluded that TCZ did not result in significant liver-related side effects [52]. On the other hand, another study reported the presence of DILI after TCZ use in combination with previous use of lopinavir/ritonavir [49], while another study by Hundt et al. proved the presence of DILI after the use of lopinavir/ritonavir, hydroxychloroquine, remdesivir, and especially, TCZ [53].

However, it is important to mention that severe DILI is very rarely a complication of TCZ administration [51] and that TCZ has a rather positive therapeutic effect when it comes to COVID-19 and the CRS. Therefore, when administering TCZ to COVID-19 patients, intense liver function monitoring is suggested, since there is always the potential of hepatotoxicity [51]. A similar profile can also be found in sarilumab, another anti-IL-6R monoclonal antibody, which is often used as an alternative to TCZ [54].

A mention should also be made regarding JAK inhibitors (baricitinib, tofacitinib, and imatinib), which were approved in many countries for treating COVID-19, as they showed significant results in reducing mortality and intubation rates [55]. There have been some cases of dose-dependent increases of liver enzymes and bilirubin during JAK inhibitor therapy, but they do not exceed 1% of the COVID-19 patients studied [6].

3.8. Antipyretics: Paracetamol or Acetaminophen

Paracetamol or acetaminophen is the drug suggested as a first-line drug for COVID-19-associated high fever and pain [6], since it has both antipyretic and analgetic effects. Paracetamol inhibits cyclooxygenases (COX-1, COX-2, and COX-3) and modulates the endocannabinoid system and the serotonergic pathways [6].

Paracetamol-induced DILI is a common cause of DILI. In adults, the average dose that causes hepatotoxicity is 12 g, and peak levels of toxicity occur 48–96 h after overdose [56]. The liver injury mechanism is direct damage that depends on the dose of paracetamol provided through acetaminophen metabolite NAPQI [6]. It is suggested that even lower doses than the ones needed for overdose can lead to the development of liver damage [6]. Moreover, patients suffering from NAFLD are more prone to developing DILI from paracetamol at lower doses than patients with a relatively healthy liver [22]. It is also worth mentioning that acetaminophen-associated DILI can be favored by an elevation in hepatic CYP2E1 [23], which is present in alcoholic patients or patients with NAFLD [23].

3.9. Other Medications

NSAIDs, also commonly used against COVID-19 [6], operate through the inhibition of cyclooxygenase (COX)-1 and -2. The most common adverse effects of NSAID therapy are gastrointestinal and renal malfunctions. However, there are reports of NSAID-induced liver damage [6]. As a matter of fact, in a cohort study, NSAIDs were responsible for over one-third of all the cases of DILI studied [57].

Colchicine is another treatment used as a COVID-19 therapy to suppress inflammation and reduce the severity of the disease's progress [4,7]. Colchicine seems to have some DILI potential, but this can be avoided by using low and regulated doses [4,58].

LMWHs are commonly used as anticoagulants to treat COVID-19 patients, since they have positive effects on reducing both mortality and morbidity [6]. At the same time, they have some adverse effects, including bleeding events, thrombocytopenia, and hepatotoxicity [6]. More specifically, LMWH is the most hepatotoxic anticoagulant used in COVID-19 therapy, with a rate of LMWH-induced liver injury of 4.3–13% [6]. When using LMWH, liver enzyme elevation usually occurs within 5 to 8 days after the initiation of heparin. After that, liver enzyme concentrations return to normal within two weeks of drug cessation [6].

Molnupiravir is an oral, antiviral drug that is highly effective when it comes to eliminating SARS-CoV-2 and viral RNA, while being quite safe. Most common side effects include headache, insomnia, and an increase in ALT, and medical professionals should be careful when administering molnupiravir to patients with hepatic dysfunction. However, it is not associated with clinically apparent liver injury [59,60].

3.10. DILI Prophylaxis and Therapy

Not much can be done to prevent DILI development, but there are some preventative measures that should be taken. Primarily, it is vital that ALT, AST, total and direct bilirubin, and albumin levels are monitored during hospitalization—especially when DILI is suspected—in order to reduce the chances of liver injury [7]. Furthermore, patients with severe COVID-19 infection and patients with pre-existing liver disease should not be administered more than two drugs at the same time or drugs that could be hepatotoxic [7]. However, clinical professionals should take into account the severity of COVID-19 disease and balance the potential positive effects of therapeutic regimens against the potential hepatotoxicity. It shall not be forgotten that severe DILI is very rare in patients with COVID-19 who have no underlying chronic liver disease [61]. When it comes to patients being treated with ongoing anti-HBV and anti-HCV drugs, their medications should not be discontinued, but they should be monitored closely [7].

There are no specific guidelines for DILI treatment during COVID-19 infection. Most of the time, treatment is not warranted, since the most beneficial measure seems to be either the discontinuation of the drug causing the DILI or alteration of its dosage [1]. This method results in recovery in 90% of the cases [6]. Given the therapeutic advantages that some of these drugs offer regarding COVID-19 infection, their discontinuation is not always easily decided upon [6]. If acute liver failure occurs; however, there is no other choice [6]. It is important to fight the virus, while also maintaining liver function [4].

4. Conclusions

Occasionally, new drugs are implicated as potential hepatotoxins that can eventually lead to DILI. Especially when it comes to COVID-19, new medications are constantly developing, thus creating new treatment possibilities that could potentially exhibit fewer adverse effects, be more hepatotoxic and detrimental, or even do both. It is a fact that most medications have undesirable side effects. In most of the cases, the DILI that occurs is not significant, and the physician in charge should be able to carefully calibrate the benefit of the drugs against their potential complications. However, it is essential to be able to detect and regulate the occasional adverse effects to an extent that eliminates deteriorating conditions.

Author Contributions: Conceptualization, E.K. and D.P.; investigation, E.K., K.P., P.P. and E.Z.; writing—original draft preparation, E.K. and K.P.; writing—review and editing, E.K., D.P., V.E.G., G.K., A.A.P., V.F. and C.S.; supervision, D.P., G.K. and C.S. All authors have read and agreed to the published version of the manuscript.

Funding: This research received no external funding.

Institutional Review Board Statement: Not applicable.

Informed Consent Statement: Not applicable.

Data Availability Statement: Not applicable.

Conflicts of Interest: The authors declare no conflict of interest.

References

1. Ortiz, G.X.; Lenhart, G.; Becker, M.W.; Schwambach, K.H.; Tovo, C.V.; Blatt, C.R. Drug-induced liver injury and COVID-19: A review for clinical practice. *World J. Hepatol.* **2021**, *13*, 1143–1153. [CrossRef] [PubMed]
2. Thakur, V.; Ratho, R.; Kumar, P.; Bhatia, S.; Bora, I.; Mohi, G.; Saxena, S.; Devi, M.; Yadav, D.; Mehariya, S. Multi-Organ Involvement in COVID-19: Beyond Pulmonary Manifestations. *J. Clin. Med.* **2021**, *10*, 446. [CrossRef] [PubMed]
3. Jothimani, D.; Venugopal, R.; Abedin, M.F.; Kaliamoorthy, I.; Rela, M. COVID-19 and the liver. *J. Hepatol.* **2020**, *73*, 1231–1240. [CrossRef]
4. Vitiello, A.; La Porta, R.; D'Aiuto, V.; Ferrara, F. The risks of liver injury in COVID-19 patients and pharmacological management to reduce or prevent the damage induced. *Egypt. Liver J.* **2021**, *11*, 1–6. [CrossRef] [PubMed]
5. Zhang, C.; Shi, L.; Wang, F.-S. Liver injury in COVID-19: Management and challenges. *Lancet Gastroenterol. Hepatol.* **2020**, *5*, 428–430. [CrossRef] [PubMed]

6. Gabrielli, M.; Franza, L.; Esperide, A.; Gasparrini, I.; Gasbarrini, A.; Franceschi, F. Liver Injury in Patients Hospitalized for COVID-19: Possible Role of Therapy. *Vaccines* **2022**, *10*, 192. [CrossRef] [PubMed]
7. Sodeifian, F.; Seyedalhosseini, Z.S.; Kian, N.; Eftekhari, M.; Najari, S.; Mirsaeidi, M.; Farsi, Y.; Nasiri, M.J. Drug-Induced Liver Injury in COVID-19 Patients: A Systematic Review. *Front. Med.* **2021**, *8*, 731436. [CrossRef]
8. D'Ardes, D.; Boccatonda, A.; Cocco, G.; Fabiani, S.; Rossi, I.; Bucci, M.; Guagnano, M.T.; Schiavone, C.; Cipollone, F. Impaired coagulation, liver dysfunction and COVID-19: Discovering an intriguing relationship. *World J. Gastroenterol.* **2022**, *28*, 1102–1112. [CrossRef]
9. Adenote, A.; Dumic, I.; Madrid, C.; Barusya, C.; Nordstrom, C.W.; Prada, L.R. NAFLD and Infection, a Nuanced Relationship. *Can. J. Gastroenterol. Hepatol.* **2021**, *2021*, 1–10. [CrossRef]
10. Vranić, L.; Radovan, A.; Poropat, G.; Mikolašević, I.; Milić, S. Non-Alcoholic Fatty Liver Disease and COVID-19–Two Pandemics Hitting at the Same Time. *Medicina* **2021**, *57*, 1057. [CrossRef]
11. Andrade, R.J.; Aithal, G.P.; Björnsson, E.S.; Kaplowitz, N.; Kullak-Ublick, G.A.; Larrey, D.; Karlsen, T.H. EASL Clinical Practice Guidelines: Drug-induced liver injury. *J. Hepatol.* **2019**, *70*, 1222–1261. [CrossRef] [PubMed]
12. Sipos, M.; Farcas, A.; Leucuta, D.; Bucsa, C.; Huruba, M.; Mogosan, C. Second-Generation Cephalosporins-Associated Drug-Induced Liver Disease: A Study in VigiBase with a Focus on the Elderly. *Pharmaceuticals* **2021**, *14*, 441. [CrossRef] [PubMed]
13. Radovanovic, M.; Dushenkovska, T.; Cvorovic, I.; Radovanovic, N.; Ramasamy, V.; Milosavljevic, K.; Surla, J.; Jecmenica, M.; Radulovic, M.; Milovanovic, T.; et al. Idiosyncratic Drug-Induced Liver Injury Due to Ciprofloxacin: A Report of Two Cases and Review of the Literature. *Am. J. Case Rep.* **2018**, *19*, 1152–1161. [CrossRef] [PubMed]
14. Teschke, R. Idiosyncratic DILI: Analysis of 46,266 Cases Assessed for Causality by RUCAM and Published From 2014 to Early 2019. *Front. Pharmacol.* **2019**, *10*, 730. [CrossRef]
15. Boeckmans, J.; Rodrigues, R.; Demuyser, T.; Piérard, D.; Vanhaecke, T.; Rogiers, V. COVID-19 and drug-induced liver injury: A problem of plenty or a petty point? *Arch. Toxicol.* **2020**, *94*, 1367–1369. [CrossRef]
16. Xu, Z.; Shi, L.; Wang, Y.; Zhang, J.; Huang, L.; Zhang, C.; Liu, S.; Zhao, P.; Liu, H.; Zhu, L.; et al. Pathological findings of COVID-19 associated with acute respiratory distress syndrome. *Lancet Respir. Med.* **2020**, *8*, 420–422. [CrossRef]
17. El-Ghiaty, M.A.; Shoieb, S.M.; El-Kadi, A.O. Cytochrome P450-mediated drug interactions in COVID-19 patients: Current findings and possible mechanisms. *Med. Hypotheses* **2020**, *144*, 110033. [CrossRef]
18. Delgado, A.; Stewart, S.; Urroz, M.; Rodríguez, A.; Borobia, A.M.; Akatbach-Bousaid, I.; González-Muñoz, M.; Ramírez, E. Characterisation of Drug-Induced Liver Injury in Patients with COVID-19 Detected by a Proactive Pharmacovigilance Program from Laboratory Signals. *J. Clin. Med.* **2021**, *10*, 4432. [CrossRef]
19. Danan, G.; Teschke, R. RUCAM in Drug and Herb Induced Liver Injury: The Update. *Int. J. Mol. Sci.* **2015**, *17*, 14. [CrossRef] [PubMed]
20. Teschke, R.; Méndez-Sánchez, N.; Eickhoff, A. Liver Injury in COVID-19 Patients with Drugs as Causatives: A Systematic Review of 996 DILI Cases Published 2020/2021 Based on RUCAM as Causality Assessment Method. *Int. J. Mol. Sci.* **2022**, *23*, 4828. [CrossRef]
21. Kamath, P.; Kamath, A.; Ullal, S.D. Liver injury associated with drug intake during pregnancy. *World J. Hepatol.* **2021**, *13*, 747–762. [CrossRef]
22. Licata, A.; Minissale, M.G.; Distefano, M.; Montalto, G. Liver injury, SARS-COV-2 infection and COVID-19: What physicians should really know? *GastroHep* **2021**, *3*, 121–130. [CrossRef] [PubMed]
23. Ferron, P.-J.; Gicquel, T.; Mégarbane, B.; Clément, B.; Fromenty, B. Treatments in Covid-19 patients with pre-existing metabolic dysfunction-associated fatty liver disease: A potential threat for drug-induced liver injury? *Biochimie* **2020**, *179*, 266–274. [CrossRef]
24. Brennan, P.N.; Cartlidge, P.; Manship, T.; Dillon, J.F. Guideline review: EASL clinical practice guidelines: Drug-induced liver injury (DILI). *Front. Gastroenterol.* **2022**, *13*, 332–336. [CrossRef] [PubMed]
25. Sun, J.; Deng, X.; Chen, X.; Huang, J.; Huang, S.; Li, Y.; Feng, J.; Liu, J.; He, G. Incidence of Adverse Drug Reactions in COVID-19 Patients in China: An Active Monitoring Study by Hospital Pharmacovigilance System. *Clin. Pharmacol. Ther.* **2020**, *108*, 791–797. [CrossRef] [PubMed]
26. Fan, Z.; Chen, L.; Li, J.; Cheng, X.; Yang, J.; Tian, C.; Zhang, Y.; Huang, S.; Liu, Z.; Cheng, J. Clinical Features of COVID-19-Related Liver Functional Abnormality. *Clin. Gastroenterol. Hepatol.* **2020**, *18*, 1561–1566. [CrossRef] [PubMed]
27. Hayashi, P.H.; Lucena, M.I.; Fontana, R.J.; Bjornsson, E.S.; Aithal, G.P.; Barnhart, H.; Gonzalez-Jimenez, A.; Yang, Q.; Gu, J.; Andrade, R.J.; et al. A revised electronic version of RUCAM for the diagnosis of DILI. *Hepatology* **2022**, *76*, 18–31. [CrossRef] [PubMed]
28. Pichler, W.J.; Tilch, J. The lymphocyte transformation test in the diagnosis of drug hypersensitivity. *Allergy* **2004**, *59*, 809–820. [CrossRef] [PubMed]
29. Cai, Q.; Huang, D.; Yu, H.; Zhu, Z.; Xia, Z.; Su, Y.; Li, Z.; Zhou, G.; Gou, J.; Qu, J.; et al. COVID-19: Abnormal liver function tests. *J. Hepatol.* **2020**, *73*, 566–574. [CrossRef]
30. Karamchandani, K.; Dalal, R.; Patel, J.; Modgil, P.; Quintili, A. Challenges in Sedation Management in Critically Ill Patients with COVID-19: A Brief Review. *Curr. Anesthesiol. Rep.* **2021**, *11*, 107–115. [CrossRef]

31. Wendel-Garcia, P.D.; Erlebach, R.; Hofmaenner, D.A.; Camen, G.; Schuepbach, R.A.; Jüngst, C.; Müllhaupt, B.; Bartussek, J.; Buehler, P.K.; Andermatt, R.; et al. Long-term ketamine infusion-induced cholestatic liver injury in COVID-19-associated acute respiratory distress syndrome. *Crit. Care* **2022**, *26*, 1–12. [CrossRef]
32. Cortes, M.G.; Robles-Diaz, M.; Stephens, C.; Ortega-Alonso, A.; Lucena, M.I.; Andrade, R.J. Drug induced liver injury: An update. *Arch. Toxicol.* **2020**, *94*, 3381–3407. [CrossRef] [PubMed]
33. Hu, P.-F.; Xie, W.-F. Corticosteroid therapy in drug-induced liver injury: Pros and cons. *J. Dig. Dis.* **2019**, *20*, 122–126. [CrossRef] [PubMed]
34. Kaur, M.; Tiwari, D.; Sidana, V.; Mukhopadhyay, K. Remdesivir-Induced Liver Injury in a COVID-Positive Newborn. *Indian J. Pediatr.* **2022**, *89*, 826. [CrossRef] [PubMed]
35. Beigel, J.H.; Tomashek, K.M.; Dodd, L.E.; Mehta, A.K.; Zingman, B.S.; Kalil, A.C.; Hohmann, E.; Chu, H.Y.; Luetkemeyer, A.; Kline, S.; et al. Remdesivir for the Treatment of COVID-19—Preliminary report. *N. Engl. J. Med.* **2020**, *383*, 1813–1826. [CrossRef]
36. Grein, J.; Ohmagari, N.; Shin, D.; Diaz, G.; Asperges, E.; Castagna, A.; Feldt, T.; Green, G.; Green, M.L.; Lescure, F.X.; et al. Compassionate Use of Remdesivir for Patients with Severe Covid-19. *N. Engl. J. Med.* **2020**, *382*, 2327–2336. [CrossRef]
37. Kulkarni, A.V.; Kumar, P.; Tevethia, H.V.; Premkumar, M.; Arab, J.P.; Candia, R.; Talukdar, R.; Sharma, M.; Qi, X.; Rao, P.N.; et al. Systematic review with meta-analysis: Liver manifestations and outcomes in COVID-19. *Aliment. Pharmacol. Ther.* **2020**, *52*, 584–599. [CrossRef] [PubMed]
38. Jorgensen, S.C.; Kebriaei, R.; Dresser, L.D. Remdesivir: Review of Pharmacology, Pre-clinical Data, and Emerging Clinical Experience for COVID-19. *Pharmacother. J. Hum. Pharmacol. Drug Ther.* **2020**, *40*, 659–671. [CrossRef]
39. Xu, L.; Liu, J.; Lu, M.; Yang, D.; Zheng, X. Liver injury during highly pathogenic human coronavirus infections. *Liver Int.* **2020**, *40*, 998–1004. [CrossRef]
40. Takahashi, T.; Luzum, J.A.; Nicol, M.R.; Jacobson, P.A. Pharmacogenomics of COVID-19 therapies. *NPJ Genom. Med.* **2020**, *5*, 1–7. [CrossRef]
41. Carothers, C.; Birrer, K.; Vo, M. Acetylcysteine for the Treatment of Suspected Remdesivir-Associated Acute Liver Failure in COVID-19: A Case Series. *Pharmacother. J. Hum. Pharmacol. Drug Ther.* **2020**, *40*, 1166–1171. [CrossRef]
42. Batteux, B.; Bodeau, S.; Gras-Champel, V.; Liabeuf, S.; Lanoix, J.; Schmit, J.; Andréjak, C.; Zerbib, Y.; Haye, G.; Masmoudi, K.; et al. Abnormal laboratory findings and plasma concentration monitoring of lopinavir and ritonavir in COVID-19. *Br. J. Clin. Pharmacol.* **2021**, *87*, 1547–1553. [CrossRef] [PubMed]
43. Cichoż-Lach, H.; Michalak, A. Liver injury in the era of COVID-19. *World J. Gastroenterol.* **2021**, *27*, 377–390. [CrossRef] [PubMed]
44. Yamazaki, S.; Suzuki, T.; Sayama, M.; Nakada, T.-A.; Igari, H.; Ishii, I. Suspected cholestatic liver injury induced by favipiravir in a patient with COVID-19. *J. Infect. Chemother.* **2021**, *27*, 390–392. [CrossRef]
45. Lin, S.-J.; Kuo, M.-L.; Hsiao, H.-S.; Lee, P.-T. Azithromycin modulates immune response of human monocyte-derived dendritic cells and CD4 + T cells. *Int. Immunopharmacol.* **2016**, *40*, 318–326. [CrossRef] [PubMed]
46. Pani, A.; Lauriola, M.; Romandini, A.; Scaglione, F. Macrolides and viral infections: Focus on azithromycin in COVID-19 pathology. *Int. J. Antimicrob. Agents* **2020**, *56*, 106053. [CrossRef]
47. Rismanbaf, A.; Zarei, S. Liver and Kidney Injuries in COVID-19 and Their Effects on Drug Therapy; a Letter to Editor. *Arch. Acad. Emerg. Med.* **2020**, *8*, e17. [CrossRef]
48. Kelly, M.; O'Connor, R.; Townsend, L.; Coghlan, M.; Relihan, E.; Moriarty, M.; Carr, B.; Melanophy, G.; Doyle, C.; Bannan, C.; et al. Clinical outcomes and adverse events in patients hospitalised with COVID-19, treated with off-label hydroxychloroquine and azithromycin. *Br. J. Clin. Pharmacol.* **2021**, *87*, 1150–1154. [CrossRef]
49. Muhović, D.; Bojović, J.; Bulatović, A.; Vukčević, B.; Ratković, M.; Lazović, R.; Smolović, B. First case of drug-induced liver injury associated with the use of tocilizumab in a patient with COVID-19. *Liver Int.* **2020**, *40*, 1901–1905. [CrossRef]
50. Kyriakopoulos, C.; Ntritsos, G.; Gogali, A.; Milionis, H.; Evangelou, E.; Kostikas, K. Tocilizumab administration for the treatment of hospitalized patients with COVID -19: A systematic review and meta-analysis. *Respirology* **2021**, *26*, 1027–1040. [CrossRef]
51. Hammond, M.; Ramersdorfer, C.; Palitzsch, K.-D.; Schölmerich, J.; Lock, G. Letales Leberversagen nach Corticosteroidtherapie bei Hepatitis-B-Carrier-Status. *DMW Dtsch. Med. Wochenschr.* **2008**, *124*, 687–690. [CrossRef] [PubMed]
52. Guaraldi, G.; Meschiari, M.; Cozzi-Lepri, A.; Milic, J.; Tonelli, R.; Menozzi, M.; Franceschini, E.; Cuomo, G.; Orlando, G.; Borghi, V.; et al. Tocilizumab in patients with severe COVID-19: A retrospective cohort study. *Lancet Rheumatol.* **2020**, *2*, e474–e484. [CrossRef] [PubMed]
53. Hundt, M.A.; Deng, Y.; Ciarleglio, M.M.; Nathanson, M.H.; Lim, J.K. Abnormal Liver Tests in COVID-19: A Retrospective Observational Cohort Study of 1,827 Patients in a Major U.S. Hospital Network. *Hepatology* **2020**, *72*, 1169–1176. [CrossRef] [PubMed]
54. Ngamprasertchai, T.; Kajeekul, R.; Sivakorn, C.; Ruenroengbon, N.; Luvira, V.; Siripoon, T.; Luangasanatip, N. Efficacy and Safety of Immunomodulators in Patients with COVID-19: A Systematic Review and Network Meta-Analysis of Randomized Controlled Trials. *Infect. Dis. Ther.* **2022**, *11*, 231–248. [CrossRef] [PubMed]
55. Limen, R.Y.; Sedono, R.; Sugiarto, A.; Hariyanto, T.I. Janus kinase (JAK)-inhibitors and coronavirus disease 2019 (Covid-19) outcomes: A systematic review and meta-analysis. *Expert Rev. Anti-infective Ther.* **2022**, *20*, 425–434. [CrossRef] [PubMed]
56. Fisher, E.S.; Curry, S.C. Evaluation and treatment of acetaminophen toxicity. *Adv. Pharmacol.* **2019**, *85*, 263–272. [CrossRef] [PubMed]

57. Licata, A.; Minissale, M.G.; Calvaruso, V.; Craxì, A. A focus on epidemiology of drug-induced liver injury: Analysis of a prospective cohort. *Eur. Rev. Med. Pharmacol. Sci.* **2017**, *21*, 112–121.
58. Vitiello, A.; Ferrara, F. Remdesivir versus ritonavir/lopinavir in COVID-19 patients. *Ir. J. Med. Sci.* **2021**, *190*, 1249–1250. [CrossRef]
59. Fischer, W.; Eron, J.J.; Holman, W.; Cohen, M.S.; Fang, L.; Szewczyk, L.J.; Sheahan, T.P.; Baric, R.; Mollan, K.R.; Wolfe, C.R.; et al. Molnupiravir, an Oral Antiviral Treatment for COVID-19. *medRxiv* **2021**. [CrossRef]
60. Law, M.F.; Ho, R.; Law, K.W.T.; Cheung, C.K.M. Gastrointestinal and hepatic side effects of potential treatment for COVID-19 and vaccination in patients with chronic liver diseases. *World J. Hepatol.* **2021**, *13*, 1850–1874. [CrossRef]
61. Pazgan-Simon, M.; Serafińska, S.; Kukla, M.; Kucharska, M.; Zuwała-Jagiełło, J.; Buczyńska, I.; Zielińska, K.; Simon, K. Liver Injury in Patients with COVID-19 without Underlying Liver Disease. *J. Clin. Med.* **2022**, *11*, 308. [CrossRef] [PubMed]

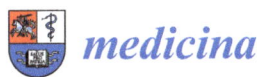

Systematic Review

Anastomotic Leak and Perioperative Outcomes of Esophagectomy for Esophageal Cancer during the COVID-19 Pandemic: A Systematic Review and Meta-Analysis

Georgios Geropoulos [1,*,†], Stavros Moschonas [2,†], Georgios Fanariotis [2], Aggeliki Koltsida [2], Nikolaos Madouros [2], Evgenia Koumadoraki [2], Kontantinos Katsikas Triantafyllidis [3], Konstantinos S. Kechagias [4], Georgios Koimtzis [5], Dimitrios Giannis [6], Athanasios Notopoulos [7], Efstathios T. Pavlidis [1] and Kyriakos Psarras [1,*]

1. Second Surgical Propedeutic Department, Hippocration Hospital, Aristotle University of Thessaloniki, 54124 Thessaloniki, Greece; pavlidis.md@gmail.com
2. Surgery Working Group, Society of Junior Doctors, 15123 Athens, Greece; mschstavros@gmail.com (S.M.); aggeliki.koltsida@gmail.com (A.K.); evgenia.koumadoraki@nhs.net (E.K.)
3. Department of Nutrition and Dietetics, Royal Marsden Hospital, London SW3 6JJ, UK; k.katsikas-triantafyllidis18@alumni.imperial.ac.uk
4. Department of Obstetrics and Gynaecology, The Hillingdon Hospitals NHS Foundation Trust, Uxbridge UB8 3NN, UK
5. Department of General Surgery, University Hospital of Wales, Cardiff and Vale University Health Board, Cardiff CF14 4XW, UK; georgios.koimtzis@wales.nhs.uk
6. Department of Surgery, Flushing Hospital Medical Center, Flushing, NY 11355, USA; dimitrisgiannhs@gmail.com
7. Department of Nuclear Medicine, Hippocration Hospital, Aristotle University of Thessaloniki, 54124 Thessaloniki, Greece; nuclearmed@ippokratio.gr

* Correspondence: georgios.geropoulos@nhs.net (G.G.); psarrask@auth.gr (K.P.)
† These authors contributed equally to this work.

Abstract: *Background and Objectives*: The coronavirus disease-2019 (COVID-19) pandemic influenced the healthcare system tremendously, as well as the number of elective surgical procedures worldwide. The aim of this study is to investigate the COVID-19 pandemic's impact on esophagectomies. *Materials and Methods*: The MEDLINE (via PubMed), Cochrane Library, and Google Scholar bibliographical databases were systematically searched. Original clinical studies investigating the outcomes of esophageal cancer surgery during the COVID-19 pandemic were deemed eligible. After exclusion criteria were applied, eight studies were considered eligible for inclusion. *Results*: Eight studies with non-overlapping populations, reporting on patients undergoing esophagectomy for resectable esophageal cancer during the COVID-19 pandemic, were included in our analysis, with a total of 18548 patients. Background characteristics for age, lung disease, smoking history as well as Body Mass Index and age were equal among the groups. The background of diabetes presented a statistically significant difference among the groups. Perioperative outcomes like reoperation rates, the length of intensive care unit stay, or readmission rates were not significantly increased during the pandemic. The 30-day readmission, and 30- and 90-day mortality were not affected either. The length of hospital stay was significantly lower in the non-pandemic period. *Conclusions*: The results of our study support the evidence that in the context of the COVID-19 pandemic, esophageal cancer operations took place safely and effectively, similarly to the standards of the non-COVID-19 era.

Keywords: esophageal cancer; COVID-19; esophagectomy; perioperative outcomes; post-operative outcomes; systematic review; meta-analysis

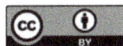

1. Introduction

The coronavirus disease-2019 (COVID-19) pandemic has significantly affected all aspects of the global healthcare system [1]. The year 2022 was marked by the emergence of the

Omicron variant as it spread and became the dominant variant worldwide. Approximately 360 million cases were reported to WHO in 2022, representing more than half of COVID-19 cases reported since the start of the pandemic, and more than during the previous two years combined [2]. The number of positive tests almost tripled in 2022, as it rose to 20% from 7% during the first two years of the pandemic. In the same year, approximately 1.2 million people are estimated to have died from COVID-19, representing one in five deaths in total. Hopefully, as WHO reported in January 2023, the number of deaths is declining overall, with between 8000 and 10,000 deaths being reported per week.

In this setting, during the first wave of the pandemic, millions of elective surgical procedures were canceled worldwide, in order to provide better care to COVID-19 patients and generally support the wider response [3]. In fact, it is estimated that, during the peak 12 weeks of disruption due to the coronavirus pandemic, the cancellation rate would be 72.3 per cent [4]. Profoundly, canceling or postponing elective surgery on this scale could potentially have an important impact on surgical patients and, consequently, catastrophic results for health systems worldwide [5]. Patients with esophageal malignancies develop multiple cancer-related complications, like pain, malnutrition, and poor performance status, with dysphagia caused by local tumor progression being one of the most frequent symptoms in patients with advanced disease. Clinicians should be alerted about dysphagia, being aware about other causes like stroke or foreign bodies, and refer to cancer centers early if other red-flag symptoms exist (weight loss, progressive dysphagia, or evidence of metastatic disease).

Furthermore, some elective surgical operations for time-sensitive cases continued, with a prioritization of patients whose underlying cancer was deemed resectable but would be at risk for progression, and patients with no other alternative effective treatment modalities. Indeed, COVID-19-free surgical pathways in both elective and major acute hospitals were established, in which elective operating rooms, critical care, and inpatient ward areas were not shared with COVID-19 patients [6]. The purpose of this study is to systematically retrospectively analyze the impact of the coronavirus pandemic on upper GI surgeries and especially on esophagectomies for esophageal cancer to assess any differences in perioperative and post-operative outcomes and delays.

2. Materials and Methods

2.1. Study Design and Inclusion/Exclusion Criteria

This systematic review and meta-analysis project was conducted according to the PRISMA (Preferred Reporting Items for Systematic Reviews and Meta-analyses) guidelines and in line with the protocol developed and agreed a priori by all authors [7]. Studies investigating esophagectomy outcomes during the COVID-19 pandemic and non-pandemic time periods were deemed eligible for analysis. As a result, two groups of patients were involved in this study: one group of patients that had an esophagectomy during the COVID-19 pandemic and one group that had an esophagectomy during the non-pandemic era. Exclusion criteria for the present systematic review were the following: (i) articles published in languages other than English; (ii) narrative, systematic, and meta-analysis reviews; (iii) case reports, errata, comments, perspectives, letters to the editor, and editorials that did not provide any primary patient data for the COVID-19 and non-COVID-19 esophagectomy period; (iv) published abstracts with no available full text; and (v) non-comparative studies (fewer than two study arms). No publication date, sample size restrictions, or any other search filters were applied.

2.2. Search Strategy

Eligible studies were identified via a search through the MEDLINE (via PubMed), Cochrane Library, and Scopus databases (end-of-search date: 1 August 2023) carried out by two independent researchers (GF and SM). The algorithm used for every search was the combination of the following keywords with all available synonyms: (esophagectomy) (esophageal cancer) AND (COVID-19). Any disagreements during the screening process were resolved by a third reviewer (GG). The reference lists and all previously published systematic reviews were thoroughly searched for missed studies eligible for inclusion based on the "snowball" methodology [8].

2.3. Data Extraction

A standardized, pre-piloted form was used for data tabulation and extraction. Two reviewers (MF and PG) extracted the data independently, and any disagreements were identified and resolved by a third reviewer (GG). We extracted the following data from the included studies: (i) study characteristics (first author, year of publication, study design, study center, country, study period, number of patients), (ii) patient characteristics (BMI, smoking, age, American Society of Anesthesiology (ASA) score of III), (iii) mortality outcomes, and iv) long-term post-operative outcomes.

2.4. Risk of Bias Assessment

The Methodological Index for Non-Randomized Studies (MINORS) was used for the risk of bias assessment of observational studies [9]. MINORS is a valid instrument designed to assess the methodological quality of non-randomized studies, whether comparative or non-comparative. MINORS' domains are scored as 0 if they are not reported, 1 when they have been reported but with inadequate details, and 2 when they have been reported while providing adequate information. The global ideal score is 16 for non-comparative studies; MINORS < 6 is considered as high risk of bias, while MINORS between 6 and 9 is considered as moderate risk of bias [9].

2.5. Statistical Analysis

The available data were handled according to the principles stated in the Cochrane Handbook [7]. Data on outcomes of interest were summarized and analyzed cumulatively. Categorical variables were reported as number of events among the total cases. Based on the extracted data, odds ratio (OR) and 95% confidence interval (CI) were calculated by means of 2×2 tables for each categorical event; OR > 1 indicated that the trait was more frequently present in the COVID-19 pandemic group. This is depicted in the forest plot for each separate variable. Between-study heterogeneity was assessed by estimating the I2 statistic. High heterogeneity was confirmed with a significance level of $p < 0.05$ and $I2 \geq 50\%$. The random-effects model was used to calculate the pooled effect when heterogeneity was high, while the fixed-effects model was used when low heterogeneity was encountered. All statistical analyses and forest plot generation were performed with the use of Reviewer Manager 5.4.1 software (Review Manager (RevMan) [Computer Program]. Version 5.4.1, Copenhagen: The Nordic Cochrane Centre, Denmark, The Cochrane Collaboration, 2020).

3. Results

A total of 150 studies were initially identified through our systematic literature search. After adjusting for duplicates, 30 of them were removed and the records of the remaining 120 underwent the screening process. As a result, 89 of them were discarded as they proved to be irrelevant, and the full text of the remaining 31 was retrieved. All these data are available in the PRISMA flow diagram (Figure 1).

Table 1 summarizes the key characteristics of the included studies. The included studies' participants ranged from 70 to 17,351, with a total of 14,301 subjects from the control group and 4247 subjects treated during the COVID-19 pandemic. The studies were conducted in various geographic regions, including Europe, the United States of America, and Japan. All studies used a case–control study design [1,10–16].

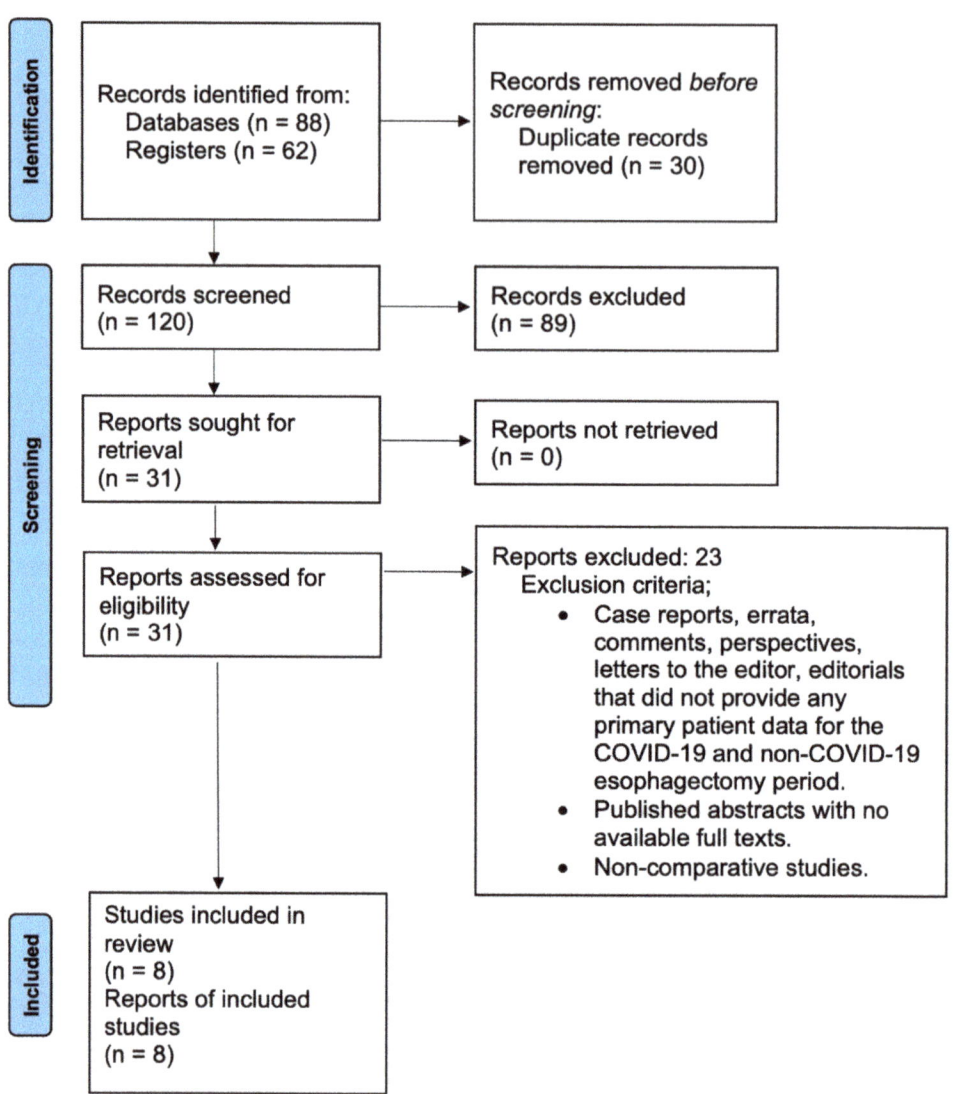

Figure 1. PRISMA 2020 flow diagram.

The overall risk of bias was low, apart from one study which was determined to have moderate risk (Table 2). The most measured outcomes were 30-day mortality, the risk of grade IV Clavien–Dindo complications, and the total length of hospital stay. However, not all studies measured the same outcomes.

Table 1. Basic characteristics of the included studies.

Author (Year)	Centre	Country	Enrolment Dates	Number of Non-Pandemic Patients (n)	Number of COVID-19 Patients (n)	Male/Female	Age (Mean ± SD)
Khan et al. (2022) [1]	The Johns Hopkins Hospital	USA	3/2019–12/2019 (Control) 3/2020–12/2020 (COVID-19)	190	117	147/43 (Control) 100/17 (COVID-19)	65.1 ± 11.3 (Control) 66.3 ± 10.8 (COVID-19)
Dolan et al. (2021) [10]	Brigham and Women's Hospital	USA	1/2019–12/2019 (Control) 3/2020–6/2020 (COVID-19)	96	37	78/18 (Control) 32/5 (COVID-19)	-
Borgstein et al. (2021) [11]	Multicenter	Netherlands, Germany, Belgium, and Sweden	10/2019–2/2020 (Control) 3/2020–5/2020 (COVID-19)	168	139	141/27 (Control) 116/23 (COVID-19)	-
Bolger et al. (2021) [12]	Irish esophageal cancer centers	Ireland	4/2019–6/2019 (Control) 4/2020–6/2020 (COVID-19)	53	45	37/16 (Control) 37/8 (COVID-19)	-
Rebecchi et al. (2020) [13]	Multicenter	Italy	3/2019–5/2019 (Control) 3/2020–5/2020 (COVID-19)	60	65		66.4 ± 3.5 (Control) 67.7 ± 6.8 (COVID-19)
Milito et al. (2022) [14]	Policlinico San Donato	Italy	3/2019–2/2020 (Control) 3/2020–10/2020 (COVID-19 first cohort) 11/2020–3/2021 (COVID-19 second cohort)	41	29	29/11 (Control) 22/7 (COVID-19)	-
Maeda et al. (2022) [15]	National Clinical Database of Japan	Japan	1/2018–4/2020 (Control) 5/2020–12/2020 (COVID-19)	13,588	3763	-	-
Miyawaki et al. (2022) [16]	National Clinical Database of Japan	Japan	4/2018–3/2020 (Control) 4/2020–3/2021 (COVID-19)	105	52	94/11 (Control) 44/8 (COVID-19)	65.9 ± 8 (Control) 69.2 ± 9.2 (COVID-19)

Table 2. Quality assessment of the included studies.

Author, Year	AIM	Inclusion of Consecutive Patients	Prospective Collection of Data	Endpoints Appropriate to the Aim of the Study	Unbiased Assessment of the Study Endpoint	Follow-Up Period Appropriate to the Aim of the Study	Loss to Follow-Up Less than 5%	Prospective Calculation of the Study Size	Total	Risk of Bias
Khan, 2022 [1]	1	2	0	2	2	2	2	0	11/16	Low
Maeda, 2022 [15]	2	2	2	2	2	2	2	0	14/16	Low
Milito, 2022 [14]	2	2	0	2	2	2	2	0	12/16	Low
Miyawaki 2022 [16]	1	2	0	2	2	2	2	0	11/16	Low
Bolger, 2021 [12]	2	2	0	2	2	0	2	0	10/16	Low
Borgstein, 2021 [11]	1	2	0	2	2	2	2	0	11/16	Low
Dolan, 2021 [10]	2	2	1	2	2	0	2	0	11/16	Low
Rebecchi, 2020 [13]	1	1	0	2	1	2	2	0	9/16	Some concerns

3.1. Baseline Patient Characteristics

Patient characteristics did not seem to have a statistically significant difference among the two groups. Patients with COPD (OR 0.92, CI 95% 0.92 to 1.49, p = 0.73, I^2 = 0%), smoking history (OR 1.40, CI 95% 0.99 to 1.98, p = 0.06, I^2 = 0%), and ASA score of III (OR 0.82, CI 95% 0.53 to 1.27, p = 0.37, I^2 = 67%) did not differ in a statistically significant manner between the groups. The patients' BMI did not fluctuate significantly (WMD 0.03, CI 95% −0.20 to 0.26, p = 0.78 I^2 = 0%); however, as was the case for the ASA score, it was only measured in two studies [1,10–12]. Age did not present a significant difference either (WMD-0.56, CI 95% −1.94 to 0.83, p = 0.08, I^2 = 53%). The only characteristic that exhibited a statistically significant difference was the incidence of diabetes (OR 0.70, CI 95% 0.49 to 0.99, p = 0.04, I^2 = 0%), as proportionally more patients with diabetes received treatment during the pandemic [1,10–14,16] (Figure 2).

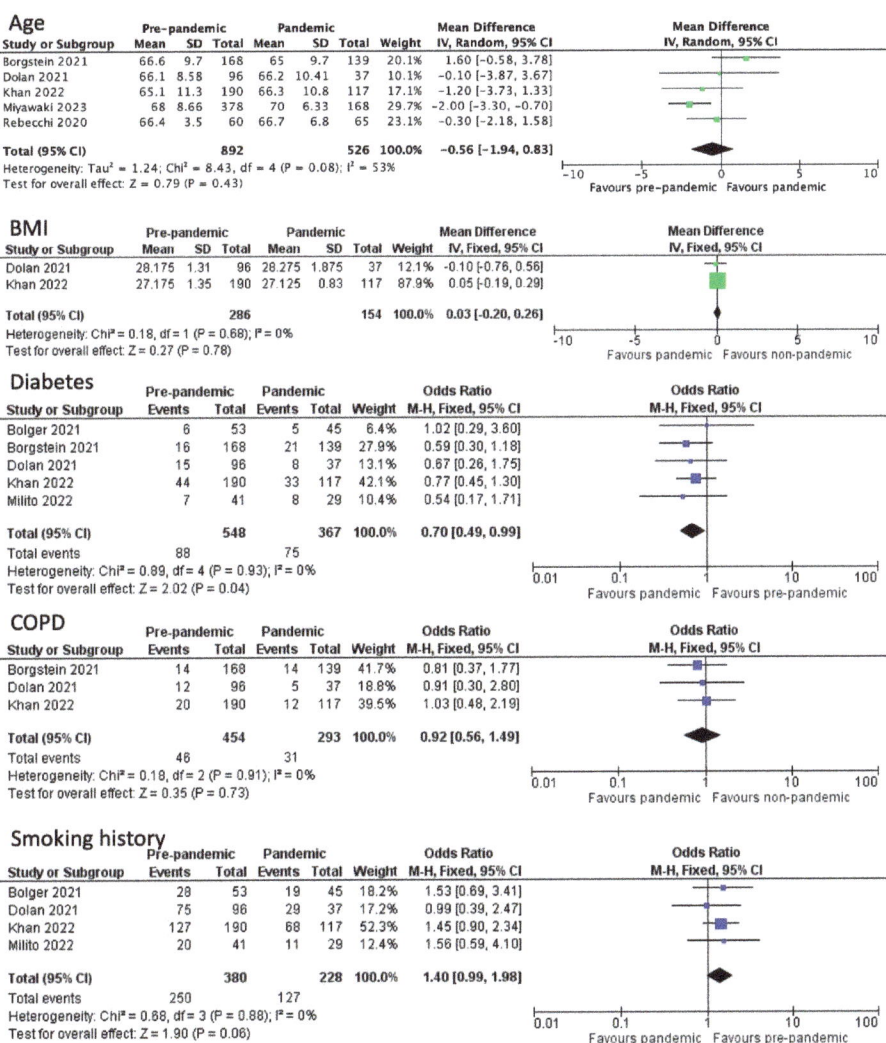

Figure 2. Patient basic characteristics [1,10–14,16].

Before moving to the post-operative outcomes, we chose to measure the proportion of patients receiving initial treatment (neoadjuvant and/or radiotherapy) in the two groups, which did not show a statistically significant difference (OR 0.98, CI 95% 0.92 to 1.04, $p = 0.47$, $I^2 = 42\%$) [1,10–12,16]. In terms of histological diagnosis, the characteristics of the tumor with regard to the prevalence of adenocarcinoma (OR 1.10, CI 95% 0.80 to 1.51, $p = 0.58$, $I^2 = 0\%$) and its location (lower third: OR 1.06, CI 95% 0.74 to 1.54, $p = 0.74$, $I^2 = 44\%$; gastroesophageal junction: OR 0.87, CI 95% 0.62 to 1.22, $p = 0.41$, $I^2 = 57\%$) did not exhibit a statistically significant difference either [1,10–12,14] (Figure 3).

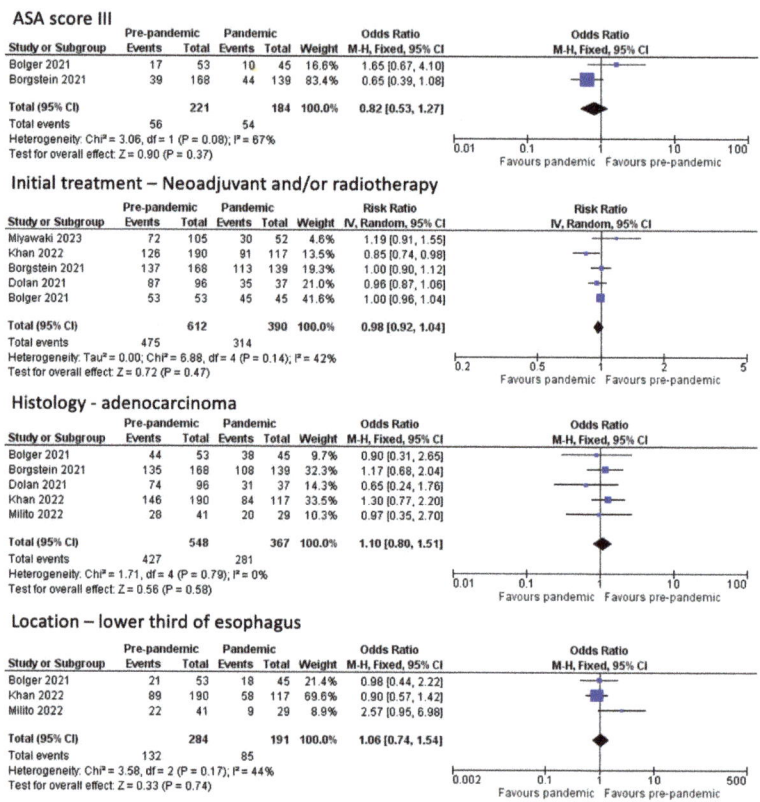

Figure 3. ASA score, treatment options, and tumor characteristics [1,10–12,14,16].

3.2. Post-Operative Outcomes

In regard to the immediate post-operative outcomes, the proportion of patients who required re-intubation (OR 0.76, CI 0.36 to 1.59, $p = 0.76$, I2 = 22%) or reoperation (OR 0.97, CI 95% 0.57 to 1.64, $p = 0.90$, $I^2 = 0\%$) showed no statistically significant difference. Similarly, the percentage of grade IV Clavien–Dindo post-operative complications (OR 0.68, CI 0.40 to 1.16, $p = 0.16$, $I^2 = 75\%$) as well as the rates of anastomotic leak (OR 0.8, CI 95% 0.41 to 1.57, $p = 0.52$ I2 = 5%) did not differ. These data are also coherent with the rates of conversion to an open surgical procedure (OR 0.67, CI 0.2 to 1.82, $p = 0.43$, $I^2 = 57\%$), which also showed no statistically significant difference (Figure 4).

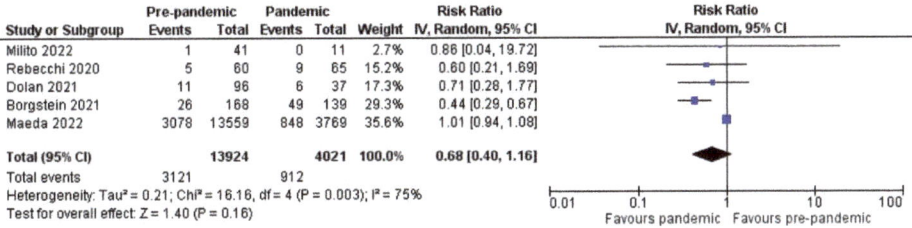
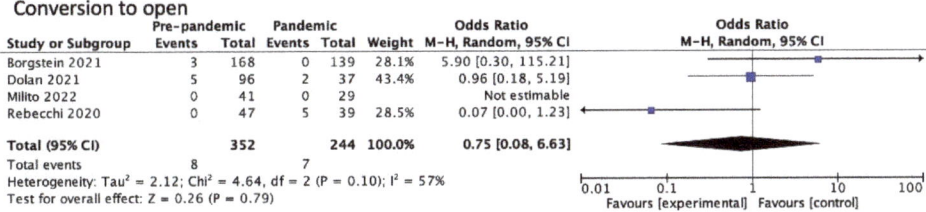

Figure 4. Immediate post-operative outcomes [1,10–15].

The effects of the immediate post-operative period carry on to the rest of the hospital stay of the patients, as the rates for ITU readmission (RR 1.29, 95% CI 0.43 to 3.90, $p = 0.65$ $I^2 = 0\%$) and the overall length of the ITU hospitalization (WMD 0.47, CI 95% -0.14 to 1.07, $p = 0.13$, $I^2 = 75\%$) had no statistically significant differentiation between the groups. However, the only measured outcome that showed statistically significant difference was the overall length of hospitalization (WMD 1.25, CI 95% 0.64 to 1.85, $p < 0.001$, $I^2 = 16\%$), where the non-pandemic group had a significantly lower overall length of hospitalization. Long-term post-operative outcomes, including the 30-day readmission (OR 0.68, CI 95% 0.41 to 1.14, $p = 0.14$, $I^2 = 0\%$), the 30-day mortality (OR 1.09, CI 95% 0.74 to 1.62, $p = 0.65$, $I^2 = 0\%$), and the 90-day mortality rates (OR 1.06, CI 95% 0.25 to 4.53, $p = 0.94$, $I^2 = 0\%$) showed no statistically significant difference (Figures 5 and 6). The funnel plot analysis of the aforementioned variables is depicted in Figures 7 and 8.

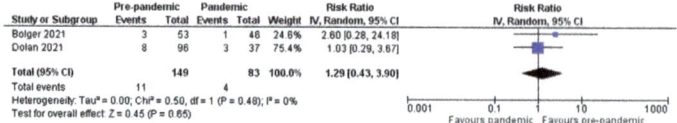
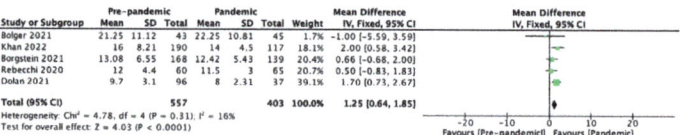
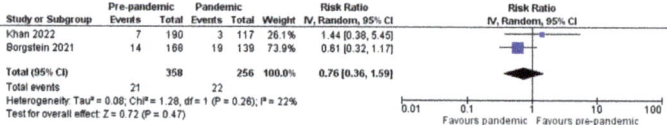
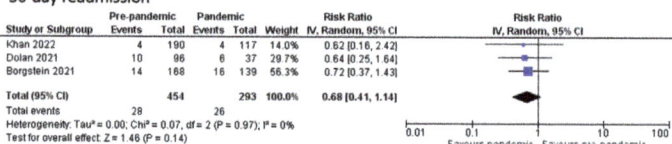

Figure 5. Perioperative outcomes [1,10–13].

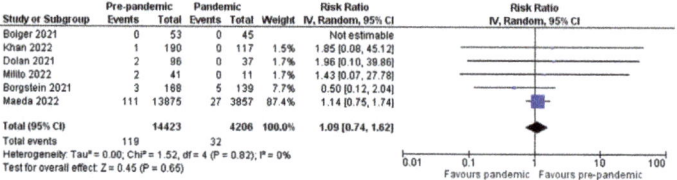
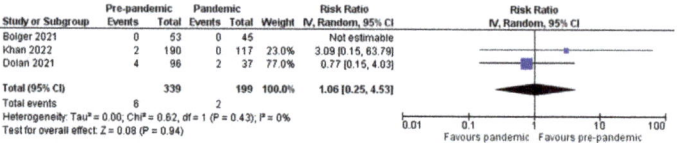

Figure 6. Readmission and mortality outcomes [1,10–12,14,15].

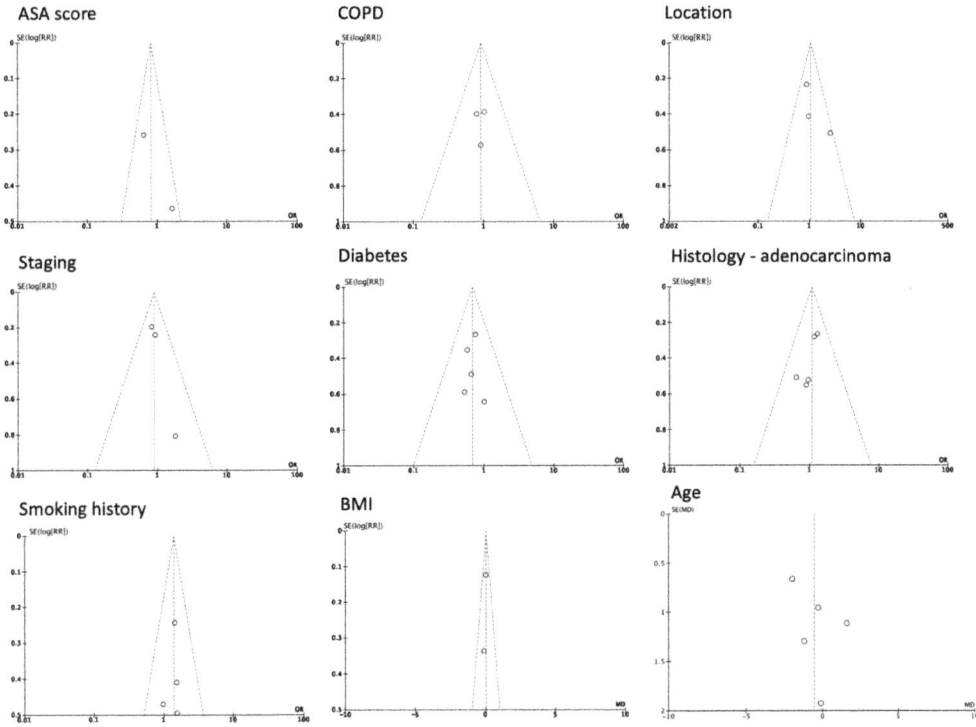

Figure 7. Funnel plots of basic patient characteristic outcomes.

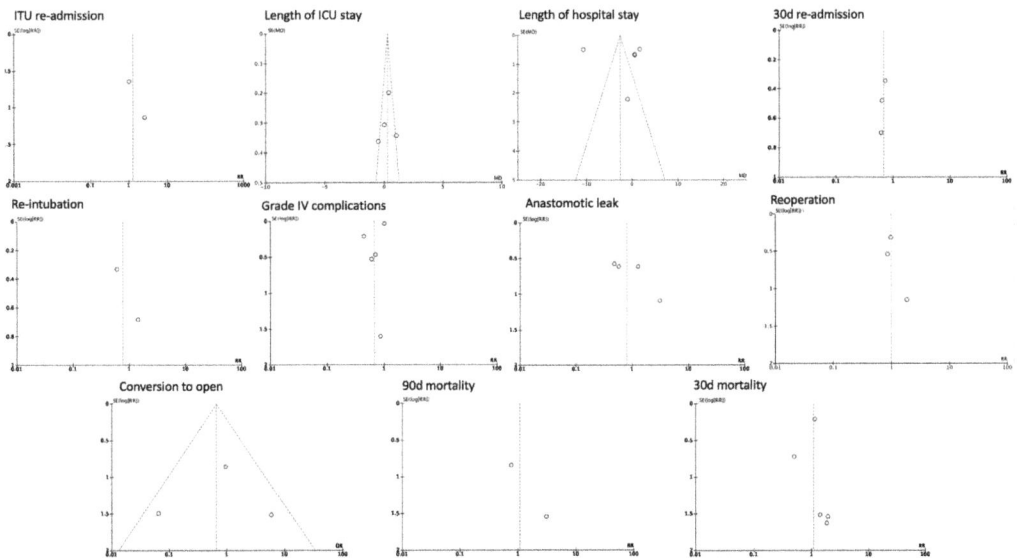

Figure 8. Funnel plots of immediate and long-term outcomes.

4. Discussion

This systematic review and meta-analysis project attempted to study the effects of the COVID-19 pandemic on patients undergoing esophagectomy. The aim of this study is to compare patient outcomes undergoing a surgical treatment of esophageal cancer during the COVID-19 pandemic versus the non-COVID-19 pandemic era. More specifically, we found that most outcomes (30-day mortality, 30-day readmission rate, 90-day mortality, the initial type of treatment offered, re-intubation, conversion to open surgical procedure, reoperation, anastomotic leak, ITU readmission, graded IV Clavien–Dindo post-operative complications, and the length of ITU hospitalization) did not differ significantly between the two groups. The length of total hospitalization as well as the diabetes were the only patient characteristics that had a statistically significant differentiation among the ones that were included in this study. These results support the fact that during the pandemic, safe esophagectomy practice could exist. It seems that policies taken by different hospitals around the world led to the safe surgical management of esophageal malignancies.

The management of esophageal cancer includes surgery, radiation therapy, chemotherapy, immunotherapy, or a combination of these treatment strategies [17]. The absence of a statistically significant difference in the type of initial therapy modalities offered for esophageal cancer patients during the COVID-19 pandemic, compared to the treatment modalities administered to another group of patients a year before the pandemic, is a strong indicator of a high-quality organizational effort and the persistence of healthcare staff to continue to provide a quality of service as close to the established standard of care as possible. While the pandemic did have a dampening effect on the activities of many surgical institutes and intensive care units, some centers for esophageal cancer modified their protocols to be able to run as a green hub [10,18]. As a result, their personnel were able to act as close as possible to the pre-pandemic standard of care. Furthermore, the similarity in esophageal cancer treatment rates before and during the COVID-19 pandemic sheds light on the prioritization that was ensured for this group of high-risk patients. All the aforementioned factors may have contributed to the fact that esophagectomy did not meet the fate of other elective procedures during the COVID-19 pandemic [19].

Basic patient characteristics (BMI, COPD, smoking history, and ASA score of III), as well as histological features (adenocarcinoma, and location at the lower third of the esophagus), did not exhibit a statistically significant difference apart from age and diabetes. In the case of chronological age, it was more common for the patients receiving surgical treatment before the pandemic to be younger. Although no clear explanation exists, a potential reason for having younger patients in the non-pandemic era may be attributed to lockdown policies where young people seek solely emergency care rather than preventive medicine. On the other hand, old people tend to have a more extensive disease at the initial diagnosis and become significantly symptomatic, so they may seek emergency care more frequently [20]. Similarly, patients with esophageal cancer and diabetes constitute a group whose physiology and characteristics play a significant part in the decision-making process for a surgical oncology operation. Combining this with the fact that the presence of diabetes acts as an independent factor for decreased pathologic complete response, as Alvarado et al. showed in a recent study, these factors could justify the prioritization of diabetic patients to receive surgical treatment for esophageal cancer [21]. However, further research is deemed necessary to clarify the age and diabetes differences presented in this study.

Adding to that, the statistical data of post-operative mortality at 30 and 90 days did not display any remarkable difference between the pre-pandemic and pandemic settings. Moreover, it is likely that the SARS-CoV-2 infection itself did not affect the early post-operative outcomes of the esophageal cancer patients undergoing esophagectomy. However, admittedly, many institutions had to implement different strategies regarding patient selection. One could raise an argument about the unknown number of patients with undiagnosed esophageal cancer who did not seek medical advice in a timely manner due to hesitancy in accessing healthcare services because of the fear of COVID-19 transmission. Thus, a group of this feeble high-risk population, perhaps, did not undergo esophageal resection even though such a population would be eligible for esophagectomy. It is possible that this phenomenon could obscure the true effect of SARS-CoV-2 infection on the post-operational prognosis of esophageal cancer patients.

While most of the outcomes that were included in this meta-analysis had no statistical significance, only the total length of hospitalization was favored during the time of the pandemic. All other metrics associated with post-operative complications (30-day mortality and readmission, 90-day mortality, the initial type of treatment offered, re-intubation, conversion to open surgical procedure, reoperation, anastomotic leak and ITU readmission, graded IV Clavien–Dindo post-operative complications, and the length of ITU hospitalization) were found to have no statistically significant difference between the groups. Our study concludes that the total length of hospital stay during the COVID-19 pandemic is significantly increased. However, other case series report a significant decrease in the length of hospital stay during the COVID-19 pandemic [22–24]. One important component of the decreased hospital stay presented by these studies could be assigned to improved infection control measures during the pandemic and the need for early discharge [25,26]. A reduced patient volume during the pandemic could have provided the chance for individualized care to patients, potentially leading to a different recovery pathway and better outcomes for the patients [1,10,27].

Nevertheless, the challenging question of whether the SARC-CoV-2 infection itself presents perioperative risks for patients undergoing esophagectomy, as no patient in the included studies contracted COVID-19 during the post-operative period, is yet to be determined. However, in the included studies, there is also no evidence that it can influence them negatively, for example via anastomotic leakage [12]. With regard to more severe complications requiring ITU readmission, re-intubation, or reoperation, they also were not noted to differentiate in a statistically significant manner between the groups. As far as re-intubation is concerned, it could be attributed to complications such as pneumonia [5], respiratory failure, or anastomotic leak, which also did not differ between the two groups, or to pre-existing factors such as respiratory disease and prolonged surgery duration. The fact that severe complications were avoided, to the point that more intensive methods of care were not administered further, proves both the non-significant changes between the populations studied and the quality of care provided. However, these results should be interpreted with caution as no patients actually had a COVID-19 infection.

It must be mentioned that our meta-analysis does have some limitations. As more and more studies continue to be published about the effects of the COVID-19 pandemic on esophagectomy outcomes, the extra data could provide a clearer view of these effects, and therefore provide us with more definitive conclusions. Moreover, the studies included were conducted in high-level institutes of specialized care for esophageal cancer. It could certainly be speculated that the COVID-19 pandemic might have had different results in other institutes, where the creation of green hubs was not possible, and the re-allocation of sources to the more critically ill COVID-19 patients was unproportionally prioritized. Furthermore, the increased hospital stay may be attributed to the fact that several hospitals implemented preoperative COVID-19 testing, with the patient remaining inpatient in quarantine while awaiting for the results. Obviously, this could increase the hospital stay in the pandemic era. This stresses the need to perform further research on whether preoperative COVID-19 or any other virology testing could take place in places other than hospitals (in home settings, for example) to reduce the hospital stay or unnecessary patient hospital visits. Our included studies varied in terms of institution origin, such as the United States of America, the United Kingdom, Italy, and Japan. This reflects the diversity of the included population and may raise the potential selection bias given. Also, there was a significant difference in the included studies' participants, where the only study with more than 1000 patients was the Maeda et al. Although the heterogeneity was low in some outcomes, the length of hospital stay and age presented high heterogeneity. So, these outcomes should be interpreted with caution while more studies with more patients are needed to achieve more unbiased results.

5. Conclusions

It has been demonstrated that during the COVID-19 pandemic, the major perioperative outcomes of operations for esophageal cancer remain unaffected. Nevertheless, safe surgical operations both for the patients and the surgeons were achieved with the appropriate systemwide policies and patient management.

Author Contributions: Conceptualization, G.G., D.G., A.N. and K.P.; methodology, S.M., G.F. and A.K.; software, G.G.; validation, G.G., G.K., K.K.T. and K.S.K.; formal analysis, G.G., K.K.T. and K.S.K.; investigation, G.G. and N.M.; resources, G.G. and K.S.K.; data curation, G.G., S.M., N.M., E.K. and G.K.; writing—original draft preparation, S.M., G.F., A.K., G.G., G.K., K.S.K. and K.K.T.; writing—review and editing, S.M., G.F., A.K., G.G., N.M. and G.K.; visualization, G.G., G.K., K.K.T. and K.S.K.; supervision, G.G., E.T.P. and K.P.; project administration, G.G. All authors have read and agreed to the published version of the manuscript.

Funding: This systematic review received no external funding.

Institutional Review Board Statement: Not applicable.

Informed Consent Statement: Not applicable.

Data Availability Statement: No new data are created.

Conflicts of Interest: The authors declare no conflict of interest.

References

1. Khan, H.; Johnson, C.; Malwankar, J.; Battafarano, R.; Yang, S.; Broderick, S.; Huang, P.; Lam, V.; Ha, J. The COVID-19 Era Is Associated With Delays in Esophageal Cancer Diagnosis and Treatment. *J. Surg. Res.* **2023**, *285*, 100–106. [CrossRef] [PubMed]
2. WHO Coronavirus (COVID-19) Dashboard. Available online: https://covid19.who.int/ (accessed on 1 June 2023).
3. Dong, E.; Du, H.; Gardner, L. An Interactive Web-Based Dashboard to Track COVID-19 in Real Time. *Lancet Infect. Dis.* **2020**, *20*, 533–534. [CrossRef] [PubMed]
4. Nepogodiev, D.; Abbott, T.E.; Ademuyiwa, A.O.; AlAmeer, E.; Bankhead-Kendall, B.K.; Biccard, B.M.; Chakrabortee, S.; Chaudhry, D.; Edwards, J.G.; El-Boghdadly, K.; et al. Projecting COVID-19 Disruption to Elective Surgery. *Lancet* **2022**, *399*, 233–234. [CrossRef] [PubMed]
5. Nepogodiev, D.; Bhangu, A.; Glasbey, J.C.; Li, E.; Omar, O.M.; Simoes, J.F.; Abbott, T.E.; Alser, O.; Arnaud, A.P.; Bankhead-Kendall, B.K.; et al. Mortality and Pulmonary Complications in Patients Undergoing Surgery with Perioperative SARS-CoV-2 Infection: An International Cohort Study. *Lancet* **2020**, *396*, 27–38. [CrossRef] [PubMed]
6. Glasbey, J.C.; Nepogodiev, D.; Simoes, J.F.; Omar, O.; Li, E.; Venn, M.L.; Abou Chaar, M.K.; Capizzi, V.; Chaudhry, D.; Desai, A.; et al. Elective Cancer Surgery in COVID-19–Free Surgical Pathways During the SARS-CoV-2 Pandemic: An International, Multicenter, Comparative Cohort Study. *J. Clin. Oncol.* **2021**, *39*, 66–78. [CrossRef] [PubMed]
7. Liberati, A.; Altman, D.G.; Tetzlaff, J.; Mulrow, C.; Gøtzsche, P.C.; Ioannidis, J.P.; Clarke, M.; Devereaux, P.J.; Kleijnen, J.; Moher, D. The PRISMA statement for reporting systematic reviews and meta-analyses of studies that evaluate healthcare interventions: Explanation and elaboration. *BMJ* **2009**, *339*, b2700. [CrossRef] [PubMed]
8. Wohlin, C. Guidelines for Snowballing in Systematic Literature Studies and a Replication in Software Engineering. In Proceedings of the 18th International Conference on Evaluation and Assessment in Software Engineering, New York, NY, USA, 13 May 2014; pp. 1–10.
9. Slim, K.; Nini, E.; Forestier, D.; Kwiatkowski, F.; Panis, Y.; Chipponi, J. Methodological index for non-randomized studies (MINORS): Development and validation of a new instrument. *ANZ J. Surg.* **2003**, *73*, 712–716. [CrossRef]
10. Dolan, D.P.; Swanson, S.J.; Lee, D.N.; Polhemus, E.; Kucukak, S.; Wiener, D.C.; Bueno, R.; Wee, J.O.; White, A. Esophagectomy for Esophageal Cancer Performed During the Early Phase of the COVID-19 Pandemic. *Semin. Thorac. Cardiovasc. Surg.* **2022**, *34*, 1075–1080. [CrossRef]
11. Borgstein, A.B.J.; Brunner, S.; Hayami, M.; Moons, J.; Fuchs, H.; Eshuis, W.J.; Gisbertz, S.S.; Bruns, C.J.; Nafteux, P.; Nilsson, M.; et al. Safety of Esophageal Cancer Surgery During the First Wave of the COVID-19 Pandemic in Europe: A Multicenter Study. *Ann. Surg. Oncol.* **2021**, *28*, 4805–4813. [CrossRef]
12. Bolger, J.C.; Donlon, N.E.; Butt, W.; Neary, C.; Al Azzawi, M.; Brett, O.; King, S.; Downey, E.; Arumugasamy, M.; Murphy, T.; et al. Successful Maintenance of Process and Outcomes for Oesophageal Cancer Surgery in Ireland during the First Wave of the COVID-19 Pandemic. *Ir. J. Med. Sci.* **2022**, *191*, 831–837. [CrossRef]

13. Rebecchi, F.; Arolfo, S.; Ugliono, E.; Morino, M.; Asti, E.; Bonavina, L.; Borghi, F.; Coratti, A.; Cossu, A.; De Manzoni, G.; et al. Impact of COVID-19 Outbreak on Esophageal Cancer Surgery in Northern Italy: Lessons Learned from a Multicentric Snapshot. *Dis. Esophagus* **2021**, *34*, doaa124. [CrossRef] [PubMed]
14. Milito, P.; Asti, E.; Resta, M.; Bonavina, L. Minimally Invasive Esophagectomy for Cancer in COVID Hospitals and Oncological Hubs: Are the Outcomes Different? *Eur. Surg.* **2022**, *54*, 98–103. [CrossRef]
15. Maeda, H.; Endo, H.; Yamamoto, H.; Miyata, H.; Munekage, M.; Taketomi, A.; Kakeji, Y.; Seto, Y.; Yoshida, K.; Yamaue, H.; et al. Effects of the COVID-19 Pandemic on Gastroenterological Surgeries in 2020: A Study Using the National Clinical Database of Japan. *Ann. Gastroenterol. Surg.* **2023**, *7*, 407–418. [CrossRef] [PubMed]
16. Miyawaki, Y.; Sato, H.; Lee, S.; Fujita, S.; Oya, S.; Sugita, H.; Hirano, Y.; Okamoto, K.; Koyama, I.; Sakuramoto, S. Impact of the Coronavirus Disease 2019 Pandemic on First-Visit Patients with Oesophageal Cancer in the First Infection Wave in Saitama Prefecture near Tokyo: A Single-Centre Retrospective Study. *Jpn. J. Clin. Oncol.* **2022**, *52*, 456–465. [CrossRef] [PubMed]
17. Harada, K.; Rogers, J.E.; Iwatsuki, M.; Yamashita, K.; Baba, H.; Ajani, J.A. Recent Advances in Treating Oesophageal Cancer. *F1000Research* **2020**, *9*, 1189. [CrossRef] [PubMed]
18. NHS England. *Specialty Guides for Patient Management during the Coronavirus Pandemic. Clinical Guide for the Management of Essential Cancer Surgery for Adults during the Coronavirus Pandemic*; NHS England and NHS Improvement: London, UK, 2020.
19. Diaz, A.; Sarac, B.A.; Schoenbrunner, A.R.; Janis, J.E.; Pawlik, T.M. Elective Surgery in the Time of COVID-19. *Am. J. Surg.* **2020**, *219*, 900–902. [CrossRef]
20. Torzilli, G.; Galvanin, J.; Viganò, L.; Donadon, M.; Montorsi, M. COVID-19: Emerging Challenges for Oncological Surgery. *Glob. Health Med.* **2020**, *2*, 197–199. [CrossRef]
21. Alvarado, C.E.; Kapcio, K.C.; Lada, M.J.; Linden, P.A.; Towe, C.W.; Worrell, S.G. The Effect of Diabetes on Pathologic Complete Response Among Patients with Esophageal Cancer. *Semin. Thorac. Cardiovasc. Surg.* **2023**, *35*, 429–436. [CrossRef]
22. Yeates, E.O.; Grigorian, A.; Schellenberg, M.; Owattanapanich, N.; Barmparas, G.; Margulies, D.; Juillard, C.; Garber, K.; Cryer, H.; Tillou, A.; et al. Decreased Hospital Length of Stay and Intensive Care Unit Admissions for Non-COVID Blunt Trauma Patients during the COVID-19 Pandemic. *Am. J. Surg.* **2022**, *224*, 90–95. [CrossRef]
23. Farroha, A. Reduction in Length of Stay of Patients Admitted to a Regional Burn Centre during COVID-19 Pandemic. *Burns* **2020**, *46*, 1715. [CrossRef]
24. Dexter, F.; Epstein, R.H.; Shi, P. Proportions of Surgical Patients Discharged Home the Same or the Next Day Are Sufficient Data to Assess Cases' Contributions to Hospital Occupancy. *Cureus* **2021**, *13*, e13826. [CrossRef] [PubMed]
25. Dexter, F.; Parra, M.C.; Brown, J.R.; Loftus, R.W. Perioperative COVID-19 Defense: An Evidence-Based Approach for Optimization of Infection Control and Operating Room Management. *Anesth. Analg.* **2020**, *131*, 37–42. [CrossRef] [PubMed]
26. Mujagic, E.; Marti, W.R.; Coslovsky, M.; Soysal, S.D.; Mechera, R.; Von Strauss, M.; Zeindler, J.; Saxer, F.; Mueller, A.; Fux, C.A.; et al. Associations of Hospital Length of Stay with Surgical Site Infections. *World J. Surg.* **2018**, *42*, 3888–3896. [CrossRef] [PubMed]
27. Maringe, C.; Spicer, J.; Morris, M.; Purushotham, A.; Nolte, E.; Sullivan, R.; Rachet, B.; Aggarwal, A. The Impact of the COVID-19 Pandemic on Cancer Deaths Due to Delays in Diagnosis in England, UK: A National, Population-Based, Modelling Study. *Lancet Oncol.* **2020**, *21*, 1023–1034. [CrossRef]

Disclaimer/Publisher's Note: The statements, opinions and data contained in all publications are solely those of the individual author(s) and contributor(s) and not of MDPI and/or the editor(s). MDPI and/or the editor(s) disclaim responsibility for any injury to people or property resulting from any ideas, methods, instructions or products referred to in the content.

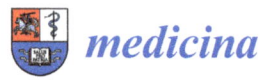

Systematic Review

The Prevalence of Gastrointestinal Bleeding in COVID-19 Patients: A Systematic Review and Meta-Analysis

Eleni Karlafti [1,2,*], Dimitrios Tsavdaris [3], Evangelia Kotzakioulafi [2], Adonis A. Protopapas [2], Georgia Kaiafa [2], Smaro Netta [3], Christos Savopoulos [2], Antonios Michalopoulos [3] and Daniel Paramythiotis [3]

[1] Emergency Department, University General Hospital of Thessaloniki AHEPA, Aristotle University of Thessaloniki, 54636 Thessaloniki, Greece
[2] 1st Propaedeutic Department of Internal Medicine, AHEPA University General Hospital, Aristotle University of Thessaloniki, 54636 Thessaloniki, Greece; evelinakotzak@hotmail.com (E.K.); adoprot@hotmail.com (A.A.P.); gdkaiafa@auth.gr (G.K.); chrisavopoulos@gmail.com (C.S.)
[3] 1st Propaedeutic Surgery Department, University General Hospital of Thessaloniki AHEPA, 54636 Thessaloniki, Greece; tsavdaris@auth.gr (D.T.); smaronetta2@gmail.com (S.N.); amichal@auth.gr (A.M.); danosprx@auth.gr (D.P.)
* Correspondence: linakarlafti@hotmail.com

Citation: Karlafti, E.; Tsavdaris, D.; Kotzakioulafi, E.; Protopapas, A.A.; Kaiafa, G.; Netta, S.; Savopoulos, C.; Michalopoulos, A.; Paramythiotis, D. The Prevalence of Gastrointestinal Bleeding in COVID-19 Patients: A Systematic Review and Meta-Analysis. *Medicina* 2023, 59, 1500. https://doi.org/10.3390/medicina59081500

Academic Editor: Claudio Gambardella

Received: 5 July 2023
Revised: 26 July 2023
Accepted: 16 August 2023
Published: 21 August 2023

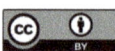

Copyright: © 2023 by the authors. Licensee MDPI, Basel, Switzerland. This article is an open access article distributed under the terms and conditions of the Creative Commons Attribution (CC BY) license (https://creativecommons.org/licenses/by/4.0/).

Abstract: *Introduction*: Severe acute respiratory syndrome coronavirus 2 caused the coronavirus disease of 2019 (COVID-19), which rapidly became a pandemic, claiming millions of lives. Apart from the main manifestations of this infection concerning the respiratory tract, such as pneumonia, there are also many manifestations from the gastrointestinal tract. Of these, bleeding from the gastrointestinal tract is a significant complication quite dangerous for life. This bleeding is divided into upper and lower, and the primary pathophysiological mechanism is the entering of the virus into the host cells through the Angiotensin-converting enzyme 2 receptors. Also, other comorbidities and the medication of corticosteroids and anticoagulants are considered to favor the occurrence of gastrointestinal bleeding (GIB). *Methods*: This systematic review was conducted following the Preferred Reporting Items for Systematic Reviews and Meta-Analyses (PRISMA) guidelines, and the studies were searched in two different databases (Scopus and PubMed) from November 2019 until February 2023. All studies that reported GIB events among COVID-19 patients were included. *Results*: 33 studies were selected and reviewed to estimate the prevalence of GIB. A total of 134,905 patients with COVID-19 were included in these studies, and there were 1458 episodes of GIB. The prevalence of GIB, in these 33 studies, ranges from 0.47% to 19%. This range of prevalence is justified by the characteristics of the COVID-19 patients. These characteristics are the severity of COVID-19, anticoagulant and other drug treatments, the selection of only patients with gastrointestinal manifestations, etc. The pooled prevalence of gastrointestinal bleeding was estimated to be 3.05%, rising to 6.2% when only anticoagulant patients were included. *Conclusions*: GIB in COVID-19 patients is not a rare finding, and its appropriate and immediate treatment is necessary as it can be life-threatening. The most common clinical findings are melena and hematemesis, which characterize upper GIB. Treatment can be conservative; however, endoscopic management of bleeding with embolization is deemed necessary in some cases.

Keywords: COVID-19; gastrointestinal bleeding

1. Introduction

Severe acute respiratory syndrome coronavirus 2 (SARS-CoV-2) is a virus that belongs to the Coronaviridae family [1]. It is a highly contagious virus, so Coronavirus disease 2019 (COVID-19), which started in Wuhan, China in December 2019, rapidly spread into a pandemic [2,3]. It is a pandemic that counts millions of deaths and more than 700 million cases. Fortunately, most cases do not require hospitalization. The virus is transmitted through aerosols and droplets, so it can easily be transmitted [2,4]. Its diagnosis can be achieved in several ways [5]. The reverse transcription polymerase chain reaction (rt-PCR) test is the gold standard technique for the diagnosis of SARS-CoV-2 [5,6], while other methods include rapid antigen SARS-CoV-2 tests [7,8]. The best way to deal with the pandemic is prevention, specifically vaccination of the population, the effectiveness of which can exceed 85% [9].

As for the symptoms of COVID-19, they appear on average 5 to 7 days after infection [3]. The most common of these are fever, fatigue, cough, and respiratory system symptoms [2,3]. However, quite often gastrointestinal symptoms also appear [2]. These include diarrhea, nausea, vomiting, anorexia, and abdominal pain [4,10]. The mechanism for GI involvement in COVID-19 is explained by the expression of angiotensin-converting enzyme 2 (ACE2) receptors in the gastrointestinal system. SARS-CoV-2 can bind to these receptors and enter host cells through the spike protein on its surface. The ability of the virus to escape from the body's immune system and the activation of the Furin protease before entering the host cell also contribute to this mechanism [2,4,10–12]. Another gastrointestinal symptom in patients suffering from COVID-19 is gastrointestinal bleeding [10,11].

Gastrointestinal bleeding (GIB) is distinguished into upper and lower bleeding with a characteristic border of the Treitz ligament. Upper gastrointestinal bleeding (UGIB) is defined as the loss of blood above the ligament of Treitz, i.e., into the duodenum, stomach, and esophagus. Its most common manifestations are melena and hematemesis [13,14]. The severity of UGIB depends on the patient's hemodynamic status, which also determines how to treat the bleeding [14]. In contrast, lower gastrointestinal bleeding (LGIB) is defined as bleeding below the ligament of Treitz [15,16]. These two types of bleeding (UGIB and LGIB) are different clinical entities and are treated differently. However, both can be a complication of COVID-19 [10].

It has not been ascertained whether the gastrointestinal bleeding in COVID-19 patients is due to the disease itself; however, it seems that the bleeding is due to other causes (e.g., perforation of a peptic ulcer or hemorrhagic gastritis) and that the pathophysiological mechanism of the COVID-19 plays a secondary role. This pathophysiological mechanism of GIB in patients with COVID-19 is explained by the entrance of SARS-CoV-2 into intestinal host cells through ACE-2 receptors that are highly expressed in gastrointestinal organs [10,11]. This entrance causes a local gastrointestinal infection that can lead to bleeding [17,18]. Bleeding can also be favored by medication against the COVID-19 infection, which usually consists of corticosteroids and anticoagulants (to treat the hypercoagulability that COVID-19 infection can cause) [19]. Finally, sepsis, pneumonia, and multiple organ failure may be causes of GIB in severely ill patients with COVID-19 [20]. This systematic review and meta-analysis aimed to determine the prevalence of GIB in patients suffering from COVID-19.

2. Materials and Methods

2.1. Study Protocol and Guidelines

This systematic review was conducted according to the Preferred Reporting Items for Systematic Reviews and Meta-Analyses (PRISMA) guidelines [21] and the MOOSE (Meta-analysis of observational studies in Epidemiology) guidelines [22]. This systematic review is registered in the Open Science Framework (OSF) with registration number: 10.17605/OSF.IO/M7PAF.

2.2. Eligibility Criteria

Eligibility criteria for this systematic review are presented in Table 1 and were defined with the PICO framework, which is the most-used model for structuring clinical questions. Observational cohort studies and cross-sectional studies with COVID-19 patients reporting GI bleeding events or prevalence of GIB were eligible for inclusion. Systematic reviews, case reports, letters to the editor, and conference abstracts were excluded.

Table 1. PICO process.

P (patient/population)	General Population
I (intervention/exposure)	COVID-19 infection
C (comparison)	-
O (outcome)	Gastrointestinal Bleeding events/prevalence of GI bleeding

2.3. Search Strategy and Selection Process

In February 2023, the systematic literature search was conducted in two databases (PubMed and Scopus). The keywords used were 'COVID-19' and 'Gastrointestinal Bleeding'. The time limit was from November 2019 (emergence of SARS-CoV-2 in China) until February 2023. The selection process was carried out by two independent reviewers (D.T. and E. Kar.) who assessed the studies' eligibility for inclusion in this systematic review using the title, abstract, and full-text evaluation in the Rayyan platform for systematic reviews. Any disagreement was solved by a third reviewer (E. Kot.).

2.4. Data Collection Process and Data Items

Data extraction was carried out by one reviewer (D.T.), and another reviewer (E. Kot.) independently checked the results. The data were extracted in a standardized Excel form. Data extraction included study details, like the author, year, country, total participants, GI bleeding prevalence, GI bleeding events, mean age of participants, and gender if mentioned. The main characteristics of each study are presented in Table 2.

2.5. Quality Assessment

Quality assessment of the included studies was performed using the Newcastle-Ottawa Quality Assessment Scale for Cohort Studies by two independent reviewers (D.T., E. Kar.). Any disagreement was solved by a third reviewer (E. Kot.). The Newcastle-Ottawa tool consists of three evaluation domains. These are the selection of participating patients, comparability, and outcomes.

Selection of participating patients includes Representativeness of the exposed cohort, Selection of the non-exposed cohort, Ascertainment of exposure, and Demonstration that the outcome of interest was not present at the start of the study. The first question regarding the representativeness of the exposed cohort is given a star when it comes to Truly or Somewhat representative. Regarding the Selection of the non-exposed cohort, a star is given if the Selection of the non-exposed cohort is drawn from the same community as the exposed cohort. To be given a star in the field Ascertainment of exposure, it must be Secure record or Structured interviews. Finally, the last star is given if there is a Demonstration that the outcome of interest was not present at the start of the study.

The 2nd domain on comparability gives two stars related to the comparability of cohorts based on design or analysis that controlled for confounders.

For the outcomes, the Assessment of the outcome and the follow-up are evaluated. For the first, a star is given if it is an Independent blind assessment or Record linkage, while, for the follow-up if it was sufficient to evaluate the results and if several of the participants submitted to it.

2.6. Statistical Analysis

Statistical analysis was performed with RevMan Software by Cochrane (v.5.3). Meta-analysis of the GI bleeding prevalence was performed using a random effects model. Heterogeneity between studies was evaluated with the I^2 and Q statistic. The investigation for publication bias was performed with the construction of funnel plots.

The statistical analysis was performed by one reviewer (D.T.), and another reviewer (E. Kot.) independently checked the results.

3. Results

3.1. Study Selection

A total of 604 studies were identified from databases PubMed and Scopus after searching the keywords 'COVID-19 patients' and 'Gastrointestinal Bleeding'. From these studies, 559 were excluded as duplicates, reviews, letters, case reports, and comments. Thus, the 93 remaining studies were screened. A total of 60 of these studies did not meet the inclusion criteria of this systematic review and were therefore excluded. Thus, 33 studies were assessed for eligibility. All 33 were included in this systematic review to estimate the prevalence of GIB in COVID-19 patients. The identification of studies for this systematic review is illustrated in the PRISMA 2020 flow chart (Figure 1). All selection stages from the initial stage to the final stage are depicted [23,24].

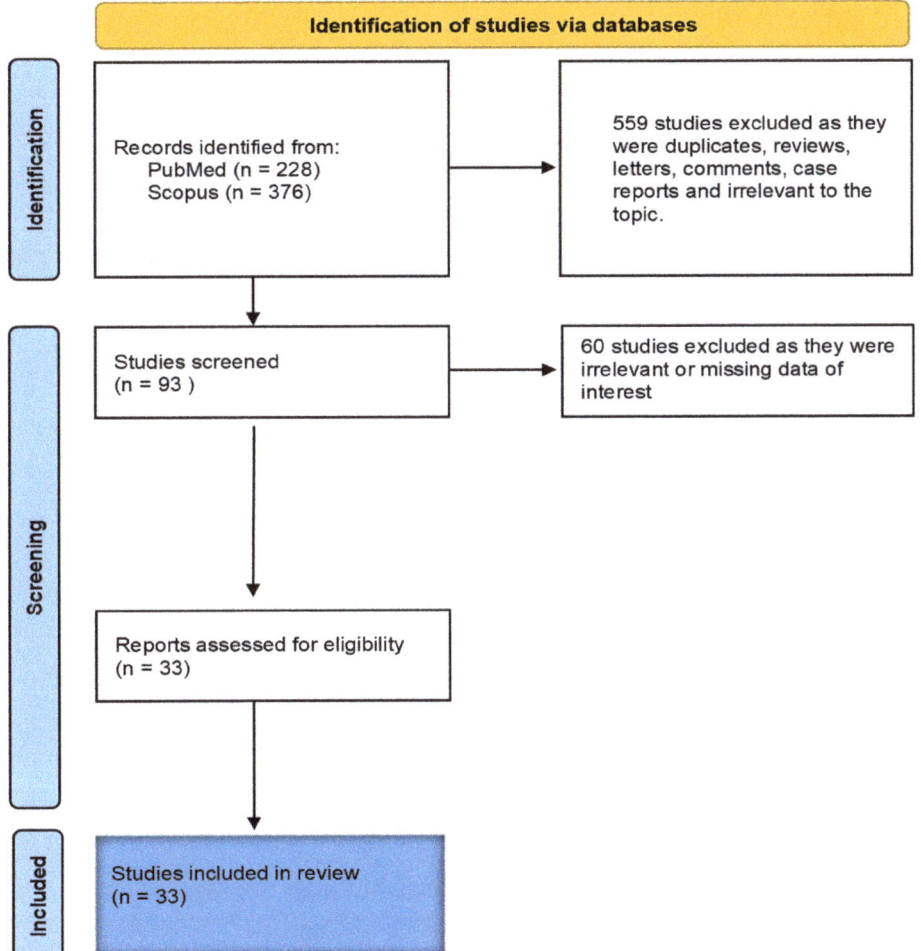

Figure 1. PRISMA flow chart summarising study identification and selection.

3.2. Study Characteristics

Among the 134,905 COVID-19 patients who participated in these 33 studies, 1458 GIB cases were reported. Of these 134,905 COVID-19 patients, the majority are male, while, at the same time, the median age exceeds 40 in all 33 studies. These studies took place in

13 different countries (China, USA, Russia, India, Brazil, Germany, Spain, Italy, Denmark, Finland, Kuwait, Romania, and Turkey). The largest study was carried out in Spain and involved 74,814 COVID-19 patients in 62 Spanish EDs. The prevalence of GIB in COVID-19 patients varies among the 33 studies and ranges from 0.47% to 19%. This large difference mainly depends on the characteristics of the COVID-19 patients who participated in the studies, which are related to taking anticoagulants or the existence of comorbidities. The characteristics of each study are presented in Table 2.

Table 2. Study Characteristics of included studies.

Study ID	Location	Total Subjects (% Male/Median Age)	Study Type	Gastrointestinal Bleeding Cases (Prevalence %)
Chen et al., 2021 [25]	China	2552 (50.4/57.8)	ORCS	40 (1.6)
Alakuş et al., 2022 [26]	Turkey	5484 (73/70.1)	ORCS	44 (0.8)
Mauro et al., 2021 [27]	Italy	4871 (78.3/75)	ORCS	23 (0.47)
Trindade et al., 2021 [28]	USA	11,158	CCS	314 (3)
Makker et al., 2021 [29]	Finland	1206 (60.8/62)	ORCS	37 (3.1)
Popa et al., 2022 [30]	Romania	1881 (66.6%)	ORCS	11 (0.58)
Prasoppokakorn et al., 2022 [31]	Thailand	6373 (65.1/69.1)	ORCS	43 (0.7)
González et al., 2022 [32]	Spain	74,814	ORCS	83 (1.11)
Lak et al., 2022 [33]	China	381 (61.4/62.6)	CS	16 (4.2)
Rosevics et al., 2021 [34]	Brazil	631(54.2/56.7)	CS	10 (1.6)
Zellmer et al., 2021 [35]	NM	5344 (57.1%)	SR	97 (1.8)
Abowali et al., 2022 [36]	USA	651 (54.2/66)	ORCS	16 (2.85)
Abulawi et al., 2022 [37]	USA	1007 (56/63)	CCS	76 (8)
Shalimar et al., 2021 [38]	India	1342 (70.8/45.8)	ORCS	24 (1.8)
Lin et al., 2020 [39]	China	95 (47/45.3)	ORCS	6 (6.3)
Shao et al., 2020 [40]	China	18 (72.2/73.5)	ORCS	1 (5.6)
Fanning et al., 2023 [41]	NM	11,969	ORCS	276 (2.3)
Zhao et al., 2021 [42]	China	368 (51.7/59)	ORCS	43 (11.7)
Martin et al., 2020 [43]	USA	987	CCS	41 (4.15)
Xiao et al., 2020 [44]	China	73 (56.1/43)	ORCS	10 (13.7)
Al-Samkari et al., 2020 [45]	USA	400	ORCS	19 (4.8)
Wan et al., 2020 [46]	China	232 (56/47)	ORCS	10 (4)
Mattioli et al., 2021 [47]	Italy	105 (58/73.7)	ORCS	2 (1.9)
Patell et al., 2020 [48]	USA	398 (52.5%)	ORCS	33 (8.29)
Bunch et al., 2021 [49]	USA	79 (65.8/71)	ORCS	2 (2.81)
Qiu et al., 2021 [50]	China	34 (71/66)	ORCS	6 (17.6)
Russell et al., 2022 [51]	Denmark	1377 (68/68)	ORCS	108 (8)
Bychinin et al., 2022 [52]	Russia	442 (43.5/78)	ORCS	9 (2)
Bonafni et al., 2022 [53]	Italy	30 (63/68.5)	ORCS	3 (10)
Abdelmohsen et al., 2021 [54]	Kuwait	30 (70/57.7)	ORCS	6 (20)
Neuberger et al., 2022 [55]	Germany	51	ORCS	2 (3.90)
Nikolay N. et al., 2022 [56]	Russia	387 (29.9/65.4)	ORCS	22 (5.7)
Demelo-Rodriguez et al., 2021 [57]	Spain	132 (47%)	ORCS	25 (19)

ORCS: Observational retrospective cohort study, CS: cross-sectional study, CCS: case-control study, SR: Survey Research.

3.3. Clinical Findings

Among the 1458 cases of GIB, 107 were manifested by melena, 79 by hematemesis and coffee ground emesis, 19 by haematochezia, 10 by severe progressive anemia and dark stool, while for the remaining cases, their manifestation and their clinical findings were not mentioned. Some of these clinical findings, such as hematemesis and melena, may have coexisted. These clinical findings are also illustrated in Figure 2.

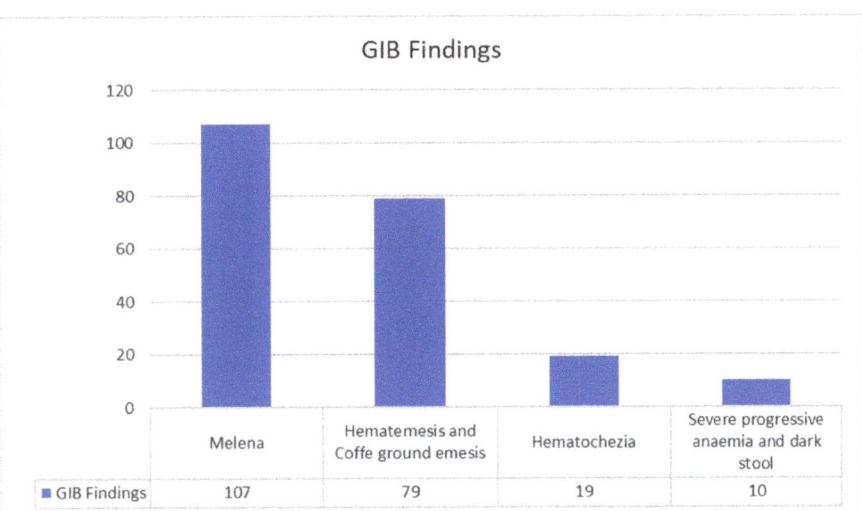

Figure 2. Clinical findings of patients with GIB. For the rest of the patients, the clinical findings are not reported.

It does not include all patients with GIB but only those clinical findings that were reported in the 33 studies. Hematemesis and melena indicate UGIB.

3.3.1. Comorbidities

Comorbidities of patients with GIB and COVID-19 were also reported. These mostly concern cardiovascular diseases and hypertension (256/1458) and diabetes (143/1458). Less common were comorbidities involving renal disease (34/1458) and malignant tumors (32/1458). Cerebrovascular disease (16/1458) and chronic respiratory disease (10/1458) were rare. Finally, various other comorbidities were reported (102/1458) such as cirrhosis and liver diseases. These comorbidities are shown in Figure 3.

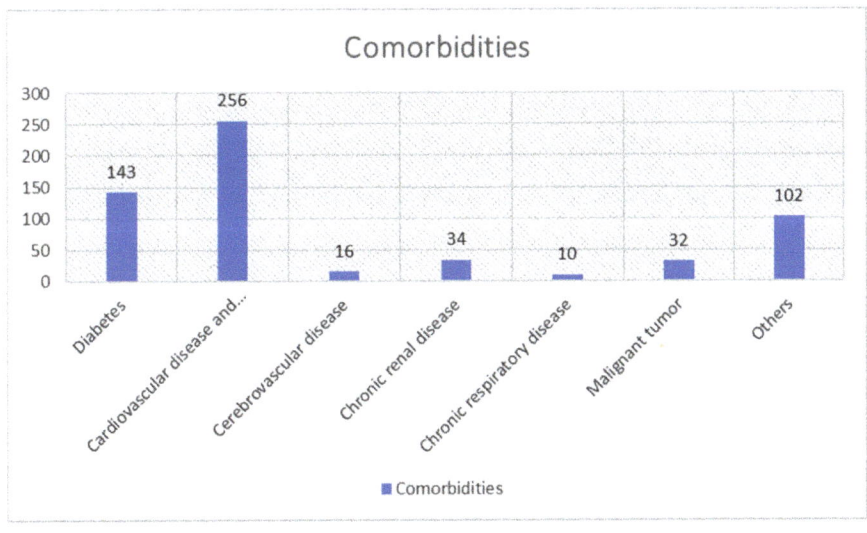

Figure 3. The main comorbidities of COVID-19 patients who experienced gastrointestinal bleeding.

Many of the above-mentioned comorbidities may have coexisted.

3.3.2. Endoscopy Characteristics

Of these 1458 cases, 286 underwent endoscopic procedures. The endoscopic findings show that the most common finding of GIB in COVID-19 patients is a gastric or duodenal ulcer (117 patients). Erosive or hemorrhagic gastritis was found in 24 patients, and variceal bleeding was also found in 24 patients. A rectal ulcer is a rarer finding and was found in 7 patients. In 55 patients, no pathological finding was found in endoscopies. The distribution of the findings is shown in Figure 4.

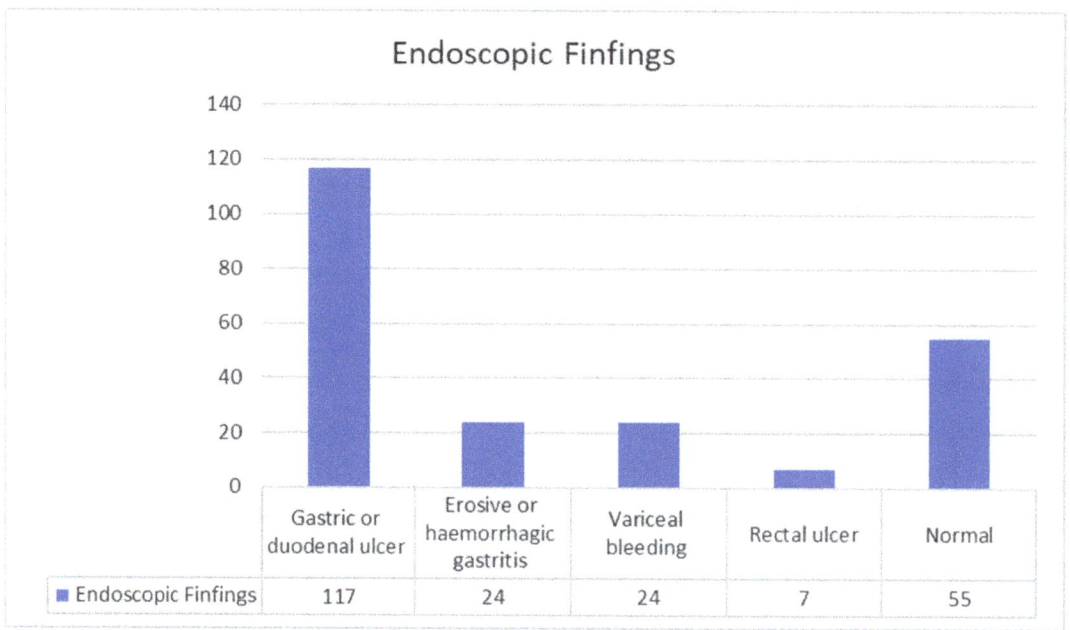

Figure 4. Findings of endoscopic procedures.

3.3.3. Laboratory Findings

A total of 19 of the 33 studies [26–29,31,32,35–38,40,42,43,45,47,51–53,57] included in this systematic review also report the laboratory findings of patients with COVID-19 who developed gastrointestinal bleeding. The Table 3 below shows these laboratory findings which are specifically hematocrit, hemoglobin, platelets, prothrombin time, INR, and d-dimers [58–61].

Table 3. Laboratory findings.

Study ID	Hematocrit (%)	Hemoglobin (g/dL)	Platelet (×10³/mm³)	Protomobin Time (s.)	International Normalized Ratio (INR)	D-Dimer (μg/mL)
Alakuş et al., 2022 [26]	22.1–33.8	7.2–11.2	88–192	13.3–15.2	1.16–1.3	1.8–2.3
Mauro et al., 2021 [27]	NM	9 (8.1–10.8)	NM	NM	NM	0.919 (0.621–2.046)
Trindade et al., 2021 [28]	NM	7.80 (6.80, 10.00)	NM	NM	NM	NM
Makker et al., 2021 [29]	NM	12 (±3)	236 (±143)	13	NM	1.034
Prasoppokakorn et al., 2022 [31]	22.5 ± 5.3	7.5 ± 1.8 (baseline: 12.6 ± 1.7)	NM	15.6 ± 5.8	1.41 ± 0.54	NM
González et al., 2022 [32]	NM	10.4 (3.2)	NM	NM	NM	NM
Zellmer et al., 2021 [35]	NM	In 22.2% of patients, it was <12	In 57.3% of patients, it was <200	NM	In 8.6% of patients, it was >1.25	NM
Abowali et al., 2022 [36]	NM	NM	NM	14.6 (13.5–16.8)	NM	0.905 (0.508–4.924)
Abulawi et al., 2022 [37]	NM	10.1 ± 2.2	NM	NM	NM	2.10 (1.17–10.16)
Shalimar et al., 2021 [38]	NM	7.2 (5.8–9.0)	90.5 (52–135)	NM	1.2 (1.2–1.4)	NM
Shao et al., 2020 [40]	NM	11.9 ± 3.2	177.50 ± 110.57	12.20 (11.50–13.40)	NM	0.49 (0.27–2.13)
Zhao et al., 2021 [42]	NM	12.6 (11.7–14.4)	161.0 (113.0–238.0)	14.2 (12.9–15.7)	NM	2.1 (0.9–11.4)
Martin et al., 2020 [43]	NM	7.5	250	NM	1.2	4.34
Al-Samkari et al., 2020 [45]	NM	NM	124 (95–154)	16.3 (14.6–17.4)	1.3 (1.2–1.4)	3.6(2.1–4.7)
Mattioli et al., 2021 [47]	NM	12.1 (10.9–13)	278.5 (186–348)	NM	1.25 (1.2–1.4)	1.4 (0.9–2.3)
Russell et al., 2022 [51]	NM	7.9 (6.7–8.6)	214 (155–290)	NM	1.1 (1.0–1.2)	1.7 (1.0–4.2)
Bychinin et al., 2022 [52]	NM	NM	189 (83.3–243)	NM	NM	0.98 (0.2–1.5)
Bonafni et al., 2022 [53]	NM	NM	239 (184–356)	NM	1.17 (1.08–1.49)	1.8 (1.1–3.1)
Demelo-Rodriguez et al., 2021 [57]	34% of patients were anemic	34% of patients were anemic	In 6% of patients, it was <100,000	In 32.5% of patients, it was >13.5 s	NM	In 94% of patients, it was >upper normal limit

NM: Not mention.

3.3.4. COVID-19 Treatments during Hospitalization in Patients with GIB

The studies in this systematic review refer to the administration of corticosteroids, anticoagulants, and proton pump inhibitors. Specifically, 112 patients received corticosteroids (administered due to hyperinflammation [62] and acute respiratory distress syndrome [63–65]). A total of 215 received anticoagulation due to coagulation disorders [66–71]. A total of 110 received low molecular weight heparin. Finally, 141 received proton pump inhibitors (to prevent bleeding in COVID-19 patients) [72,73]. These results are shown in Table 4 and concern only the incidents reported in the studies and not all patients.

Table 4. Treatment of COVID-19 patients who experienced GIB.

COVID-19 Treatments during Hospitalization in Patients with GIB	
Corticosteroids	112
Anticoagulant and antiplatelet therapy	215
LMWH	110
PPI	141

LMWH: Low Molecular Weight Heparin, PPI: Proton Pump Inhibitors.

3.3.5. Outcomes

Regarding outcomes, 119 patients were admitted to the intensive care unit, while 107 COVID-19 patients were intubated with mechanical ventilation. A total of 40 patients were discharged from the hospital, while 218 patients died. Finally, 16 rebleeding patients were reported. Outcomes are presented in Figure 5. These deaths were not solely due to gastrointestinal bleeding but to the general aggravated condition of the patients and the co-complications of the disease such as respiratory failure.

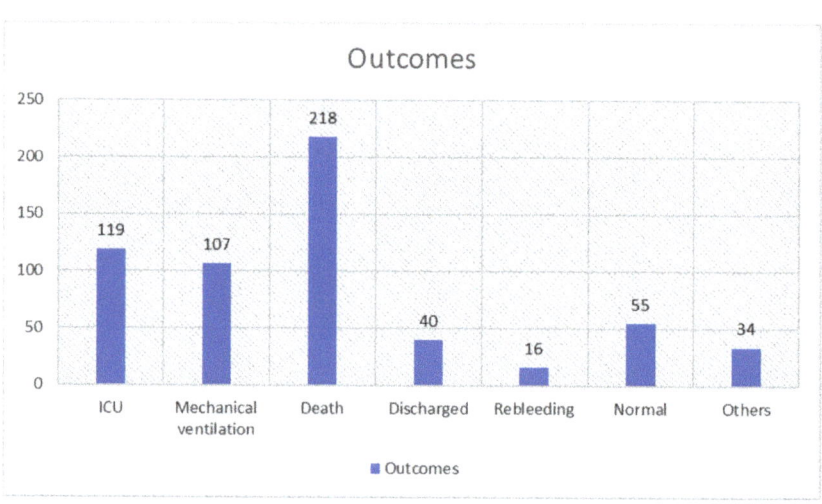

Figure 5. Outcomes of COVID-19 patients with GIB.

3.4. Quality Assessment

Quality assessment of the included studies was performed using the Newcastle-Ottawa Quality Assessment Scale for Cohort Studies by two independent reviewers (D.T., E. Kar.). The results are listed in Table 5. In the studies in our systematic review, the majority did not use a non-exposed cohort for this and were not given a star in the selection domain. All studies were evaluated with good methodological quality except for Shao et al., 2020 [40] which was considered fair quality.

Table 5. Quality Assessment.

Study ID	Selection				Comparability	Outcome			Total Quality
	Representativeness of the Exposed Cohort	Selection of the Non-Exposed Cohort	Ascertainment of Exposure	Demonstration that Outcome of Interest was not Present at the Start of the Study	Comparability of Cohorts on the Basis of the Design or Analysis Controlled for Confounders	Assessment of Outcome	Was Follow-Up Long enough for Outcomes to Occur	Adequacy of Follow-Up of Cohorts	
Abdelmohsen et al., 2021 [54]	*		*	*	**	*	*	*	8/9 GOOD
Abowali et al., 2022 [36]	*		*	*	**	*	*	*	8/9 GOOD
Abulawi et al., 2022 [37]	*		*	*	**	*	*	*	8/9 GOOD
Alakuş et al., 2022 [26]	*		*	*	**	*	*	*	8/9 GOOD
Al-Samkari et al., 2020 [45]	*		*	*	**	*	*	*	8/9 GOOD
Bonfini et al., 2022 [53]	*		*	*	**	*	*	*	8/9 GOOD
Bunch et al., 2021 [49]	*		*	*	**	*	*	*	8/9 GOOD
Bychinin et al., 2022 [52]	*		*	*	**	*	*	*	8/9 GOOD
Chen et al., 2021 [25]	*		*	*	**	*	*	*	8/9 GOOD
Fanning et al., 2023 [41]	*		*	*	**	*	*	*	8/9 GOOD
González et al., 2022 [32]	*	*	*	*	**	*	*	*	9/9 GOOD
Lak et al., 2022 [33]	*		*	*	**	*	*	*	8/9 GOOD
Lin et al., 2020 [39]	*		*	*	**	*	*	*	8/9 GOOD
Makker et al., 2021 [29]	*		*	*	**	*	*	*	8/9 GOOD
Martin et al., 2020 [43]	*		*	*	**	*	*	*	8/9 GOOD
Mattioli et al., 2021 [47]	*	*	*	*	**	*	*	*	9/9 GOOD
Mauro et al., 2021 [27]	*		*	*	**	*	*	*	8/9 GOOD
Neuberger et al., 2022 [55]	*		*	*	**	*	*	*	8/9 GOOD
Nikolay N. et al., 2022 [56]	*		*	*	**	*	*		7/9 GOOD
Patell et al., 2020 [48]	*		*	*	**	*	*	*	8/9 GOOD
Popa et al., 2022 [30]	*	*	*	*	**	*	*	*	9/9 GOOD
Prasoppokakorn et al., 2022 [31]	*		*	*	**	*	*	*	8/9 GOOD
Qiu et al., 2021 [50]	*	*	*	*	**	*	*	*	9/9 GOOD

Table 5. Cont.

Study ID	Selection				Comparability	Outcome			Total Quality
	Representativeness of the Exposed Cohort	Selection of the Non-Exposed Cohort	Ascertainment of Exposure	Demonstration that Outcome of Interest was not Present at the Start of the Study	Comparability of Cohorts on the Basis of the Design or Analysis Controlled for Confounders	Assessment of Outcome	Was Follow-Up Long enough for Outcomes to Occur	Adequacy of Follow-Up of Cohorts	
Rosevics et al., 2021 [34]	*		*	*	**	*	*	*	8/9 GOOD
Russell et al., 2022 [51]	*		*	*	**	*	*	*	8/9 GOOD
Shalimar et al., 2021 [38]	*		*	*	**	*	*	*	8/9 GOOD
Shao et al., 2020 [40]			*	*	**	*			5/9 FAIR*
Trindade et al., 2021 [28]	*		*	*	**	*	*	*	8/9 GOOD
Wan et al., 2020 [46]	*		*	*	**	*	*	*	8/9 GOOD
Xiao et al., 2020 [44]	*		*	*	**	*	*	*	8/9 GOOD
Zellmer et al., 2021 [35]	*		*	*	**	*	*	*	8/9 GOOD
Zhao et al., 2021 [42]	*		*	*	**	*	*	*	8/9 GOOD

3.5. Meta-Analysis Results

The pooled prevalence was estimated at 3.05% (2.58–3.52, 95%CI), but with high heterogeneity (I^2 96%). The forest plot of the pooled prevalence is presented in Figure 6. Below is illustrated the forest plot and the funnel plot where the prevalence ratio and the standard error are distinguished, while random effects were used to estimate the pooled prevalence. Funnel plot is presented in Figure 7.

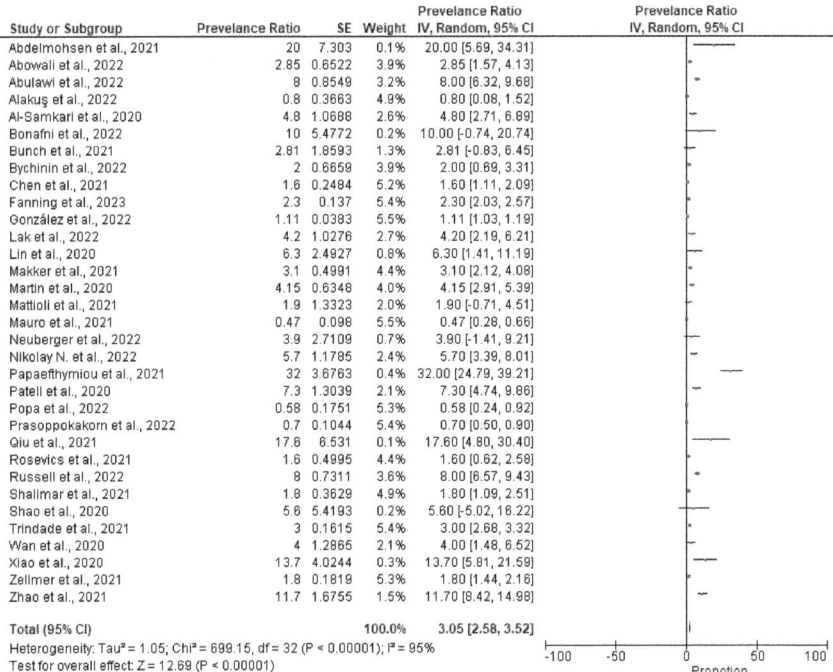

Figure 6. Forest plot of the pooled prevalence.

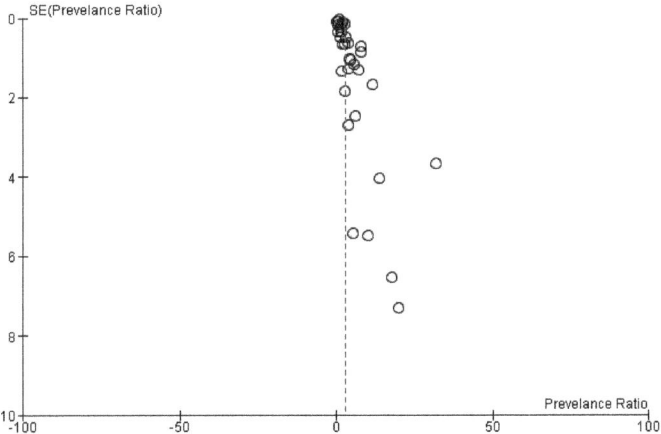

Figure 7. Funnel plot of publication bias.

Subgroup Analysis

Subgroup (1) According to Treatment

Subgroup analysis was performed based on treatment. In 9 of the 33 studies in this systematic review, patients on anticoagulation or antiplatelet therapy were included. It seems that the use of anticoagulants or antiplatelet agents increases the risk of bleeding, with results also increasing the prevalence of gastrointestinal bleeding in these studies. However, even after removing these studies, the overall prevalence is estimated at 2.69% (2.20–3.17, 95%CI) quite close to the value of 3.05% which is in the total number of COVID-19 patients. The forest plot and the funnel plot show the prevalence distribution, the ratio, and the standard error. On the contrary, the total prevalence in these 9 studies is estimated at 6.2% (3.16–9.25, 95%CI). This value highlights the increased prevalence in patients on anticoagulation or antiplatelet therapy. Heterogeneity did not differ or was reduced in the subgroup analysis. Results are presented in Figures 8 and 9. Despite this increased prevalence in anticoagulation-treated COVID-19 patients, a causal relationship between anticoagulants and gastrointestinal bleeding cannot be confirmed due to lack of data.

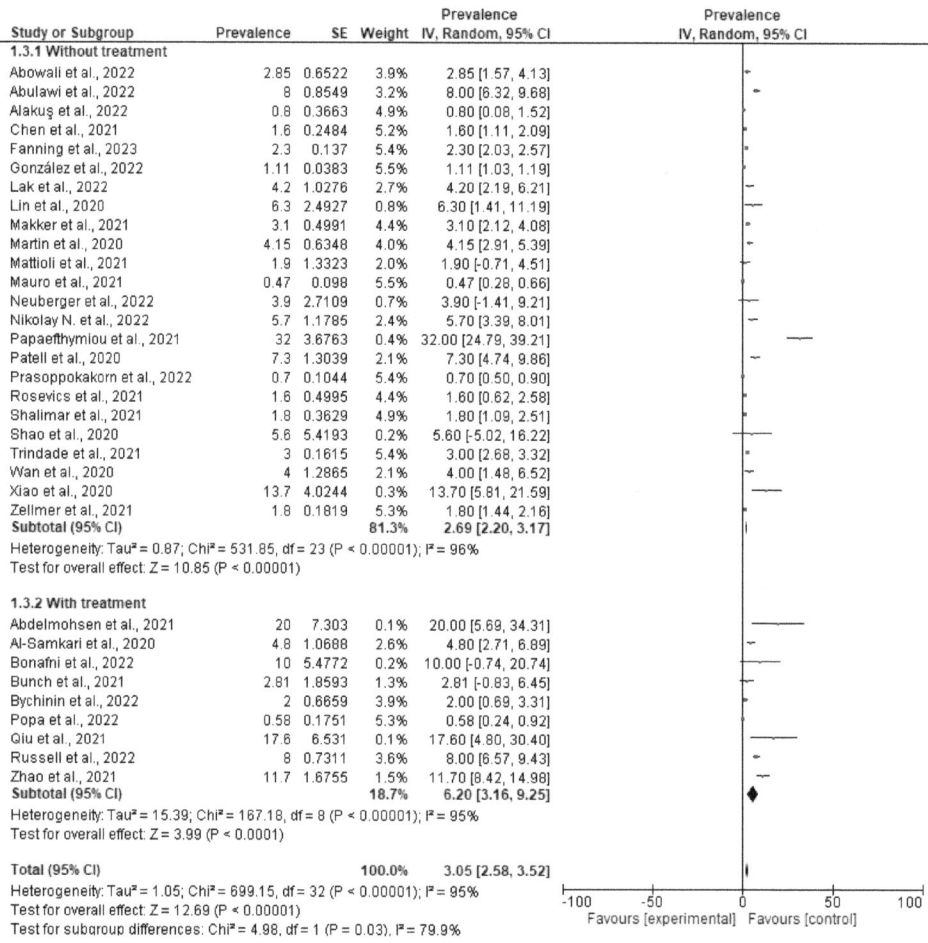

Figure 8. Forest plot of subgroup analysis based on treatment.

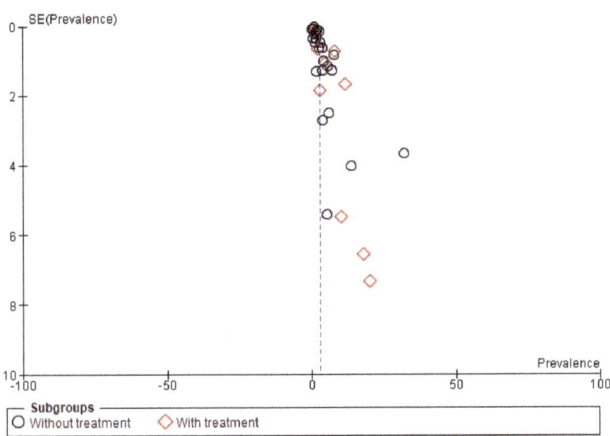

Figure 9. Funnel plot of publication bias on studies included in the subgroup (1) analysis.

Subgroup (2) According to Location of Bleeding

In 17 of the 33 studies [26–31,34,35,37,38,43,44,48,53–56] in the meta-analysis, upper or lower gastrointestinal bleeding could be distinguished. Thus, it was possible to distinguish the prevalence of GI bleeding into the upper and lower gastrointestinal tract into two subgroups. A total of 15 studies reported the prevalence of upper gastrointestinal bleeding, resulting in a pooled prevalence equal to 1.78% [1.32, 2.24, 95% CI]. Accordingly, 8 studies report the prevalence of lower gastrointestinal bleeding and give a pooled prevalence equal to 0.69% [0.30, 1.09, 95% CI] or 1%. Thus, it is understood that upper gastrointestinal bleeding is a more common complication of COVID-19 than lower gastrointestinal bleeding, a fact that is also confirmed by the clinical findings. The results are visible in Figures 10 and 11.

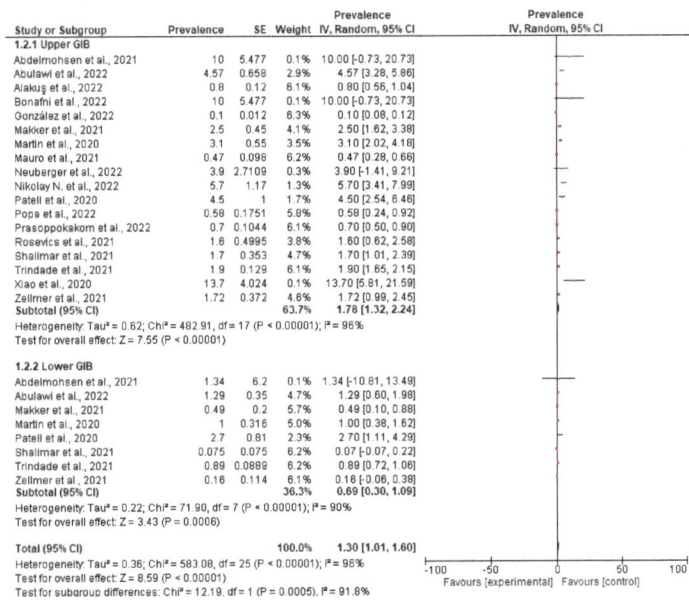

Figure 10. Forest plot of subgroup analysis according to the location of bleeding.

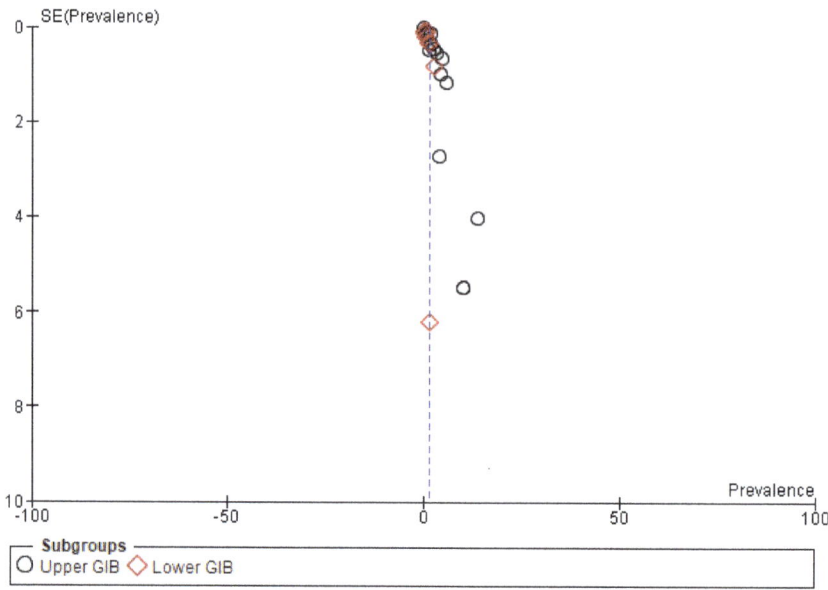

Figure 11. Funnel plot of publication bias on studies included in the subgroup (2) analysis.

3.6. Publication Bias

Publication bias was performed with the construction of funnel plots which are presented in Figures 7 and 9. The funnel plots showed asymmetry which is evidence for publication bias.

4. Discussion

In this systematic review, 33 studies were included that addressed the risk of GIB in COVID-19 patients. A total of 134,905 patients with COVID-19 participated in them, of which 1458 presented GIB. However, the prevalence of GIB differed between the studies, with the lowest value of 0.47% and the highest reaching 19%. The prevalence of GIB is influenced by several factors. It was found to be higher in studies involving COVID-19 patients on anticoagulation factors or in patients with gastrointestinal disturbances. In contrast, in studies involving patients with COVID-19 without signs of gastrointestinal involvement or in studies where the sample of patients was very large, the prevalence of GIB ranged up to 5%. Even this percentage, however, is quite significant, especially if the dangerousness of the situation is considered.

Our findings from the meta-analysis showed that the pooled prevalence of gastrointestinal bleeding is 3.05%. The 95% confidence interval of the prevalence ranges between 2.58 and 3.52, while the heterogeneity is high, reaching 96%. This percentage ranks gastrointestinal bleeding among the important complications of COVID-19, but not among the most common. However, due to the seriousness of this complication, it should be treated with caution. These percentages increase even more, reaching 6.2% (3.16–9.25, 95%CI) in patients receiving anticoagulant or antiplatelet treatment. This treatment is very common in COVID-19 patients due to the coagulopathy caused by the virus. Therefore, in patients under treatment, any symptom suggestive of gastrointestinal bleeding should be investigated, as well as gastrointestinal bleeding, and included in the differential diagnosis of various complications.

The guidelines suggest that patients presenting with GIB should undergo endoscopy within twenty-four hours, for diagnostics and therapeutic purposes [74]. However, COVID-

19 patients are a different case as they are at greater risk due to pneumonia. Also, the intubation of many COVID-19 patients is another obstacle in performing endoscopy. Finally, the risk of transmission of SARS-CoV-2 increases during such operations [75]. For this reason, the endoscopic approach to patients must be conducted with great care as long as the conditions allow it. If endoscopy is not possible, then conservative treatment is preferred. This is based on taking proton pump inhibitors, and antibiotics, while this can be enhanced by taking somatostatin and terlipressin [76,77]. Finally, fresh frozen plasma (FFP), packed red blood cells, and intravenous fluid resuscitation are administered [38].

Of the 1458 cases, 286 underwent endoscopic procedures. Gastrointestinal endoscopic procedures include esophagogastroduodenoscopy, colonoscopy, and capsule endoscopy. Esophagogastroduodenoscopies were performed in the majority of those 286 cases, as in most cases the bleeding was in the upper gastrointestinal tract. Of the 286 endoscopies, 54 had a therapeutic purpose. The endoscopic treatment of bleeding includes various techniques; the most commonly performed are injectable solutions, hemostatic substances with local action, mechanical methods, elastic rings, hemostatic knots, stapling mechanisms, or cauterization. If these fail, surgical treatment is indicated. The success of these mechanisms depends on various factors such as age, hematemesis, oligemic shock, low hematocrit, as well as other concomitant diseases [78–80]. Of the injectable solutions, adrenaline is preferred. Clips are used on endoscopically visible bleeding vessels. Elastic rings are preferred in variceal bleeding, while hemostatic knots are preferred in polypectomy bleeding.

In the era of COVID-19, therefore, a decrease in endoscopies was observed [81,82]. However, in some cases it was deemed necessary to perform endoscopy to manage GIB. These cases mainly involved males, with an increased body mass index, anticoagulant treatment, and multiple comorbidities [83,84]. However, complications due to COVID-19 in these patients led to reduced 30-day survival, with an odds ratio of 0.25 [85]. Despite reduced survival, no increase in major rebleeding was found [85]. Taking all this into account, the risks of these interventions may outweigh the benefits [84]. In addition, cases have been reported in which GIB in COVID-19 patients was self-limiting without the need for any additional intervention [86]. Finally, increased intensive care unit stays and intubations were observed for COVID-19 cases undergoing endoscopies for the management of GIB [87].

Abnormalities in normal laboratory values are also seen in COVID-19 patients with gastrointestinal bleeding. The drop in hemoglobin is evident, reaching up to the value of 7.2 g/dL, while the normal value in males is between 13.5 and 17.5 g/dL, but in females is 11.5–15.5 g/dL. The platelets appear to be in the lower normal limits, and in some cases, they are slightly reduced. Normally they should be within the range of $140–400 \times 10^3/\text{mm}^3$. Prothrombin time and INR are indicators of the body's coagulation capacity and are used as an initial control test to detect deficiencies of one or more coagulation factors (factors II, V, VII, X) as well as to monitor patients under anticoagulant therapy [60]. These seem slightly affected while finally the d-dimers (soluble fibrin degradation product) [61] were in the majority of cases above normal values. The changes in these values are due to a combination of bleeding, COVID-19, and the anticoagulant treatment that many of these patients are under.

Therefore, the outcomes of GIB in COVID-19 patients differ from non-COVID-19 patients. This difference is recorded in the stay in the intensive care units (ICU), in the use of corticosteroid drugs, intubation, as well as in the causes of death, as these mainly concern the respiratory due to the COVID-19 infection [88–90]. No differences are observed in hemoglobin, in the administration of blood and crystalloid solutions, and the rate of rebleeding. Also, the etiology of the bleeding and its clinical findings do not differ [89,90]. Finally, during the period of COVID-19, a significant decrease was observed in the number of patients coming to the hospital with GIB, which is attributed to their unwillingness to visit the hospital, due to COVID-19 [91,92]. In general, the causative agents of gastrointestinal bleeding differ slightly from the causes blamed for gastrointestinal bleeding in COVID-19 patients. In both cases, the main cause of upper digestive bleeding is peptic ulcer, followed by gastritis, duodenitis, varicocele, and esophagitis [93]. A common causative agent in non-COVID-19 patients of upper gastrointestinal bleeding is Mallory-Weis syndrome [93,94]. The etiology is more varied when it comes to bleeding from the lower gastrointestinal tract. In non-COVID-19 patients, bleeding is primarily due to diverticular disease, polyps, neoplasms, and inflammatory bowel disease [16].

Regarding mortality from GIB, 218 deaths were reported in these 33 studies involving COVID-19 patients with GIB. However, the majority of deaths is not due to the bleeding itself but due to the COVID-19 infection. About 10 were directly due to GIB. Chen et al. suggest that GIB is an independent prognostic indicator of the composite endpoint and death [25]. These findings are also supported by Popa et al [30]. Popa et al. also suggest that the administration of anticoagulants does not affect mortality. [30] Additionally, Patell et al. report an increase in mortality in patients with active cancer who suffer from COVID-19 and experience bleeding episodes [48].

An also frequently reported finding from these studies concerns the increased risk of GIB in critically and seriously ill COVID-19 patients [25,27,34,42–44,50,52,53,55]. In particular, the risk of bleeding increases in patients who require admission to an intensive care unit or are already in it, in patients on mechanical ventilation, and patients with severe COVID-19 pneumonia. Also, Zhao et al. state that in seriously ill patients the risk of hidden GIB increases, possibly due to stress-related mucosal disease (SRMD) [42]. This can be seen during gastroscopy and was observed in 2.6% of patients with GIB admitted to the ICU [95,96]. Neuberger et al. also observed in vivo that severe disease of COVID-19 may be associated with duodenal SARS-Cov-2 infection, severe duodenitis, and subsequent bleeding complications [55,97]. Laboratory findings indicating an increased risk of ICU admission are elevated D-dimers and ferritin and low platelet count [51,57]. Finally, Al-Samkari et al. state that in severe COVID-19 patients, bleeding is major, with a worse prognosis [45]. These data explain why Mauro et al., where only non-ICU patients participated, calculated the lowest prevalence of GIB in COVID-19 patients (0.47%) [27].

The most common cause of lower GIB was found to be a rectal ulcer. However, Martin et al. stress that intrarectal catheters are another cause of LGIB. These are catheters that reduce the risk of perianal skin breakdown, while at the same time reduce healthcare workers' exposure and the risk of hospital-acquired infections. These made them especially valuable in the COVID-19 pandemic. However, necrosis caused by pressure ischemia increases the risk of GIB, and this should be seriously considered before their use [43,98–100].

Patients suffering from COVID-19 often present with hyper-inflammation [62]. This hyper-inflammation is treated with the use of corticosteroids. Corticosteroids may also help treat COVID-related acute respiratory distress syndrome (ARDS) [63–65]. Of the 33 clinical studies used in this systematic review, many cases of COVID-19 patients who developed GIB while receiving corticosteroids were reported. However, the most important treatment in hospitalized COVID-19 patients that appears to be associated with the occurrence of GIB is the administration of anticoagulants [66,67]. It has been found that disturbances in the balance of vasodilator and vasoconstrictor angiotensin as well as the cytokines of sepsis caused by COVID-19 result in coagulation disorders. Up to 50% of COVID-19 patients will develop coagulopathies. [66–71] The treatment of them is based on the administration of anticoagulants and mainly low molecular weight heparin. Venous thromboembolic episodes (VTE) are very common in COVID-19 patients and may coexist with bleeding. Prophylactic treatment for venous thromboembolic events is based on anticoagulant treatment, which appears to increase the risk of bleeding, mainly gastrointestinal [101]. Despite the higher prevalence of gastrointestinal bleeding in COVID-19 patients who are under anticoagulant treatment, their association cannot be confirmed due to the lack of data about the percentage use of anticoagulants in COVID-19 patients without GI bleeding. Finally, cases of administration of proton pump inhibitors, which are administered to patients with gastric ulcers at high risk of GIB, were reported. Proton pump inhibitors have been shown to contribute significantly to the prevention of bleeding in patients on anticoagulation or antiplatelet therapy [72,73]. These patient amounts are the ones reported, as not all studies reported the treatment given to the patients.

Demelo-Rodriguez et al. included only patients receiving standard, intermediate, or therapeutic doses of VTE prophylaxis. Despite this, it appeared that the prevalence of GIB was not affected by the dose of the received treatment of anticoagulation [57]. It has also been found that prophylactic heparin treatment in COVID-19 patients reduces the need for cardiorespiratory support as well as increased survival in non-severe patients. Unfortunately, these do not apply to seriously ill patients [102,103]. Norepinephrine and ventilatory support are associated with thrombotic events, the most common of which is deep vein thrombosis [52].

Mauro et al., proposed an algorithm (Figure 12) for the management of GIB in COVID-19 patients, especially upper. According to him, first, the hemodynamic status of the patient is controlled. Then, it is judged whether the patient needs respiratory support. Then, if the patient is at low risk, endoscopy can be performed to manage the bleeding within 24 h. Otherwise, in seriously ill patients, the degree of severity is judged according to the presence of hematemesis or not [27]. According to Wan et al., the presence of diarrhea may also indicate the severity of the infection and the need for non-mechanical ventilation [46,104]. Finally, imaging findings may also be useful in diagnosing GIB. In particular, in severe COVID-19 patients, it is considered very important to perform a CT scan when there are signs that indicate the existence of bleeding [53]. In Abdelmohsen et al., the most frequent indication for a CT scan was abdominal distension [54].

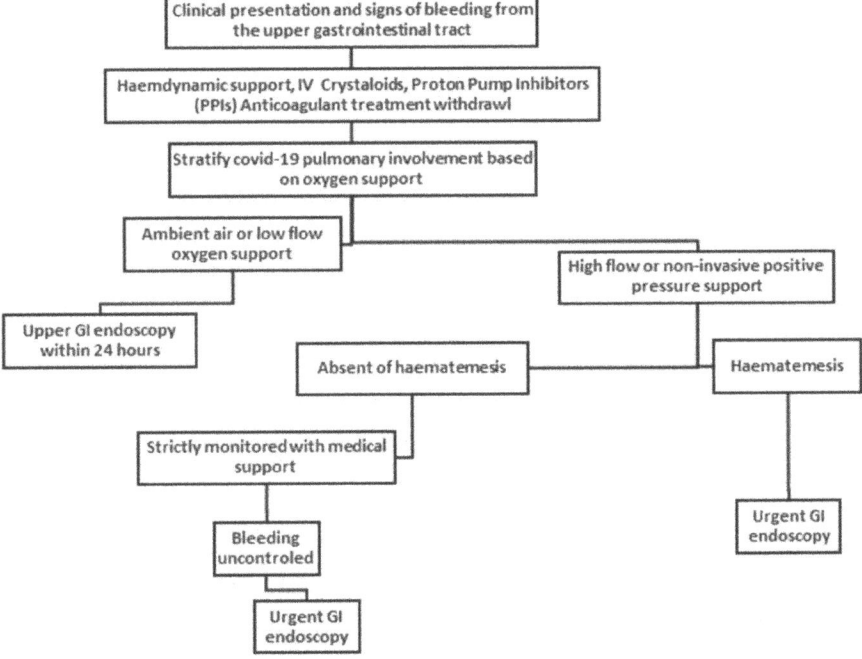

Figure 12. Management of upper gastrointestinal bleeding based on the algorithm proposed by Mauro et al. [27].

The meta-analysis of Marasco et al. estimated the overall prevalence of GIB in COVID-19 patients. This prevalence was estimated at 5%. The distribution of upper and lower bleeding was also calculated. In particular, 76.6% of the bleeding concerned the upper gastrointestinal system, while the rest concerned the lower [105]. This meta-analysis reviews only 10 observational studies and therefore only 91,887 cases of COVID-19. In contrast, the current systematic review included 33 studies and 134,905 cases of COVID-19.

Further research needs to be conducted on the safety of endoscopies in COVID-19 patients. It is also necessary to clarify how exactly GIB occurs in COVID-19 patients and whether it is caused directly by the infection or indirectly.

This meta-analysis has several strengths and limitations. Firstly, the updated literature search that includes newly published studies is the main strength compared to others. What is more, we followed a protocol for the literature search according to PRISMA guidelines. Furthermore, we conducted a subgroup analysis based on the presence of treatment or not. However, this research has some limitations. One of them is the absence of double-blind randomized studies, as only observational studies were found in the available literature. The small availability of studies on the subject, however, gives this systematic review strength, as it facilitates the synthesis of the results while simultaneously reducing the possibility of error.

5. Conclusions

In conclusion, COVID-19 patients show quite frequent gastrointestinal symptoms. Of them, GIB in COVID-19 patients is not the most common, as symptoms such as diarrhea, nausea, vomiting, and abdominal pain prevail. However, it occurs in a significant percentage and is one of the most important and dangerous complications in COVID-19 patients, where in some cases it requires urgent treatment and can even lead to death. Upper gastrointestinal bleeding is more common than lower, and the most common clinical findings are melena and hematemesis. Treatment and management of bleeding are based on either medication or endoscopic interventions such as embolization, while self-healing of bleeding is not uncommon.

Author Contributions: Conceptualization, E.K. (Eleni Karlafti), G.K., C.S., A.M. and D.P.; methodology, E.K. (Evangelia Kotzakioulafi); software, D.T.; validation, E.K. (Eleni Karlafti), D.T., E.K. (Evangelia Kotzakioulafi) and S.N.; formal analysis, E.K. (Evangelia Kotzakioulafi) and D.T.; investigation, E.K. (Eleni Karlafti), D.T., S.N. and A.A.P.; resources, D.P., A.M. and C.S.; data curation, D.T. and S.N.; writing—original draft preparation, D.T., E.K. (Eleni Karlafti) and E.K. (Evangelia Kotzakioulafi); writing—review and editing, E.K. (Eleni Karlafti), D.T., E.K. (Evangelia Kotzakioulafi), A.A.P., G.K., C.S., A.M. and D.P.; visualization, E.K. (Evangelia Kotzakioulafi) and D.T.; supervision, C.S., G.K., A.M. and D.P.; project administration, C.S., G.K., A.M. and D.P. All authors have read and agreed to the published version of the manuscript.

Funding: This systematic review received no external funding.

Institutional Review Board Statement: Not applicable.

Informed Consent Statement: Not applicable.

Data Availability Statement: No new data are created.

Conflicts of Interest: The authors declare no conflict of interest.

References

1. Leao, J.C.; Gusmao, T.P.d.L.; Zarzar, A.M.; Filho, J.C.L.; de Faria, A.B.S.; Silva, I.H.M.; Gueiros, L.A.M.; Robinson, N.A.; Porter, S.; Carvalho, A.d.A.T. Coronaviridae—Old friends, new enemy! *Oral Dis.* **2022**, *28*, 858–866. [CrossRef]
2. Wiersinga, W.J.; Rhodes, A.; Cheng, A.C.; Peacock, S.J.; Prescott, H.C. Pathophysiology, Transmission, Diagnosis, and Treatment of Coronavirus Disease 2019 (COVID-19). *JAMA* **2020**, *324*, 782. [CrossRef] [PubMed]
3. Shi, Y.; Wang, G.; Cai, X.-P.; Deng, J.-W.; Zheng, L.; Zhu, H.-H.; Zheng, M.; Yang, B.; Chen, Z. An overview of COVID-19. *J. Zhejiang Univ. Sci. B* **2020**, *21*, 343–360. [CrossRef] [PubMed]
4. Salian, V.S.; Wright, J.A.; Vedell, P.T.; Nair, S.; Li, C.; Kandimalla, M.; Tang, X.; Porquera, E.M.C.; Kalari, K.R.; Kandimalla, K.K. COVID-19 Transmission, Current Treatment, and Future Therapeutic Strategies. *Mol. Pharm.* **2021**, *18*, 754–771. [CrossRef] [PubMed]
5. Kevadiya, B.D.; Machhi, J.; Herskovitz, J.; Oleynikov, M.D.; Blomberg, W.R.; Bajwa, N.; Soni, D.; Das, S.; Hasan, M.; Patel, M.; et al. Diagnostics for SARS-CoV-2 infections. *Nat. Mater.* **2021**, *20*, 593–605. [CrossRef]

6. D'Cruz, R.J.; Currier, A.W.; Sampson, V.B. Laboratory Testing Methods for Novel Severe Acute Respiratory Syndrome-Coronavirus-2 (SARS-CoV-2). *Front. Cell Dev. Biol.* **2020**, *8*, 468. [CrossRef] [PubMed]
7. Peeling, R.W.; Heymann, D.L.; Teo, Y.-Y.; Garcia, P.J. Diagnostics for COVID-19: Moving from pandemic response to control. *Lancet* **2022**, *399*, 757–768. [CrossRef]
8. Karlafti, E.; Tsavdaris, D.; Kotzakioulafi, E.; Kaiafa, G.; Savopoulos, C.; Netta, S.; Michalopoulos, A.; Paramythiotis, D. The Diagnostic Accuracy of SARS-CoV-2 Nasal Rapid Antigen Self-Test: A Systematic Review and Meta-Analysis. *Life* **2023**, *13*, 281. [CrossRef]
9. Sharif, N.; Alzahrani, K.J.; Ahmed, S.N.; Dey, S.K. Efficacy, Immunogenicity and Safety of COVID-19 Vaccines: A Systematic Review and Meta-Analysis. *Front. Immunol.* **2021**, *12*, 714170. [CrossRef]
10. Kariyawasam, J.C.; Jayarajah, U.; Riza, R.; Abeysuriya, V.; Seneviratne, S.L. Gastrointestinal manifestations in COVID-19. *Trans. R Soc. Trop. Med. Hyg.* **2021**, *115*, 1362–1388. [CrossRef]
11. Jin, B.; Singh, R.; Ha, S.E.; Zogg, H.; Park, P.J.; Ro, S. Pathophysiological mechanisms underlying gastrointestinal symptoms in patients with COVID-19. *World J. Gastroenterol.* **2021**, *27*, 2341–2352. [CrossRef] [PubMed]
12. Anka, A.U.; Tahir, M.I.; Abubakar, S.D.; Alsabbagh, M.; Zian, Z.; Hamedifar, H.; Sabzevari, A.; Azizi, G. Coronavirus disease 2019 (COVID-19): An overview of the immunopathology, serological diagnosis and management. *Scand J. Immunol.* **2021**, *93*, e12998. [CrossRef] [PubMed]
13. Owensby, S.; Taylor, K.; Wilkins, T. Diagnosis and Management of Upper Gastrointestinal Bleeding in Children. *J. Am. Board Fam. Med.* **2015**, *28*, 134–145. [CrossRef] [PubMed]
14. Kamboj, A.K.; Hoversten, P.; Leggett, C.L. Upper Gastrointestinal Bleeding: Etiologies and Management. *Mayo Clin. Proc.* **2019**, *94*, 697–703. [CrossRef] [PubMed]
15. Aoki, T.; Hirata, Y.; Yamada, A.; Koike, K. Initial management for acute lower gastrointestinal bleeding. *World J. Gastroenterol.* **2019**, *25*, 69–84. [CrossRef] [PubMed]
16. Hawks, M.K.; Svarverud, J.E. Acute Lower Gastrointestinal Bleeding: Evaluation and Management. *Am. Fam. Physician* **2020**, *101*, 206–212.
17. Ye, Q.; Wang, B.; Zhang, T.; Xu, J.; Shang, S. The mechanism and treatment of gastrointestinal symptoms in patients with COVID-19. *Am. J. Physiol.-Gastrointest. Liver Physiol.* **2020**, *319*, G245–G252. [CrossRef]
18. Dioscoridi, L.; Giannetti, A.; Massad, M.; Forti, E.; Pugliese, F.; Cintolo, M.; Bonato, G.; Rosa, R.; Mutignani, M. A 'double-hit' damage mechanism can explain self-limited GI bleeding in COVID-19 pneumonia. *Gastrointest Endosc.* **2021**, *93*, 1192–1193. [CrossRef]
19. Sarkar, M.; Madabhavi, I.V.; Quy, P.N.; Govindagoudar, M.B. COVID-19 and coagulopathy. *Clin. Respir. J.* **2021**, *15*, 1259–1274. [CrossRef]
20. Cook, D.; Guyatt, G. Prophylaxis against Upper Gastrointestinal Bleeding in Hospitalized Patients. *N. Engl. J. Med.* **2018**, *378*, 2506–2516. [CrossRef]
21. Liberati, A.; Altman, D.G.; Tetzlaff, J.; Mulrow, C.; Gotzsche, P.C.; Ioannidis, J.P.A.; Clarke, M.; Devereaux, P.J.; Kleijnen, J.; Moher, D. The PRISMA statement for reporting systematic reviews and meta-analyses of studies that evaluate healthcare interventions: Explanation and elaboration. *BMJ* **2009**, *339*, b2700. [CrossRef] [PubMed]
22. Brooke, B.S.; Schwartz, T.A.; Pawlik, T.M. MOOSE Reporting Guidelines for Meta-analyses of Observational Studies. *JAMA Surg.* **2021**, *156*, 787. [CrossRef] [PubMed]
23. Page, M.J.; McKenzie, J.E.; Bossuyt, P.M.; Boutron, I.; Hoffmann, T.C.; Mulrow, C.D.; Shamseer, L.; Tetzlaff, J.M.; Akl, E.A.; Brennan, S.E.; et al. The PRISMA 2020 statement: An updated guideline for reporting systematic reviews. *BMJ* **2021**, *372*, n71. [CrossRef] [PubMed]
24. Page, M.J.; Moher, D.; Bossuyt, P.M.; Boutron, I.; Hoffmann, T.C.; Mulrow, C.D.; Shamseer, L.; Tetzlaff, J.M.; Akl, E.A.; Brennan, S.E.; et al. PRISMA 2020 explanation and elaboration: Updated guidance and exemplars for reporting systematic reviews. *BMJ* **2021**, *372*, n160. [CrossRef] [PubMed]
25. Chen, H.; Tong, Z.; Ma, Z.; Luo, L.; Tang, Y.; Teng, Y.; Yu, H.; Meng, H.; Peng, C.; Zhang, Q.; et al. Gastrointestinal Bleeding, but Not Other Gastrointestinal Symptoms, Is Associated with Worse Outcomes in COVID-19 Patients. *Front. Med.* **2021**, *8*, 759152. [CrossRef] [PubMed]
26. Alakuş, Ü. Upper gastrointestinal system bleedings in COVID-19 patients: Risk factors and management / A retrospective Cohort Study. *Turk. J. Trauma Emerg. Surg.* **2021**, *28*, 762–768. [CrossRef] [PubMed]
27. Mauro, A.; De Grazia, F.; Lenti, M.V.; Penagini, R.; Frego, R.; Ardizzone, S.; Savarino, E.; Radaelli, F.; Bosani, M.; Orlando, S.; et al. Upper gastrointestinal bleeding in COVID-19 inpatients: Incidence and management in a multicenter experience from Northern Italy. *Clin. Res. Hepatol. Gastroenterol.* **2021**, *45*, 101521. [CrossRef] [PubMed]
28. Trindade, A.J.; Izard, S.; Coppa, K.; Hirsch, J.S.; Lee, C.; Satapathy, S.K. Gastrointestinal bleeding in hospitalized COVID-19 patients: A propensity score matched cohort study. *J. Intern. Med.* **2021**, *289*, 887–894. [CrossRef]
29. Makker, J.; Mantri, N.; Patel, H.K.; Abbas, H.; Baiomi, A.; Sun, H.; Choi, Y.; Chilimuri, S.; Nayudu, S.K. The Incidence and Mortality Impact of Gastrointestinal Bleeding in Hospitalized COVID-19 Patients. *Clin. Exp. Gastroenterol.* **2021**, *14*, 405–411. [CrossRef]

30. Popa, P.; Iordache, S.; Florescu, D.N.; Iovanescu, V.F.; Vieru, A.; Barbu, V.; Bezna, M.-C.; Alexandru, D.O.; Ungureanu, B.S.; Cazacu, S.M. Mortality Rate in Upper Gastrointestinal Bleeding Associated with Anti-Thrombotic Therapy Before and During Covid-19 Pandemic. *J. Multidiscip. Healthc.* **2022**, *15*, 2679–2692. [CrossRef]
31. Prasoppokakorn, T.; Kullavanijaya, P.; Pittayanon, R. Risk factors of active upper gastrointestinal bleeding in patients with COVID-19 infection and the effectiveness of PPI prophylaxis. *BMC Gastroenterol.* **2022**, *22*, 465. [CrossRef] [PubMed]
32. González, R.G.; Jacob, J.; Miró, Ò.; Llorens, P.; Jiménez, S.; del Castillo, J.G.; Burillo-Putze, G.; Martín, A.; Martín-Sánchez, F.J.; Lamberechts, J.G.; et al. Incidence, Clinical Characteristics, Risk Factors, and Outcomes of Upper Gastrointestinal Bleeding in Patients With COVID-19. *J. Clin. Gastroenterol.* **2022**, *56*, e38–e46. [CrossRef] [PubMed]
33. Lak, E.; Sheikholeslami, S.; Ghorbi, M.; Shafei, M.; Yosefi, H. Association between gastrointestinal symptoms and disease severity in patients with COVID-19 in Tehran City, Iran. *Gastroenterol. Rev.* **2022**, *17*, 52–58. [CrossRef]
34. Rosevics, L.; Fossati, B.S.; Teixeira, S.; de Bem, R.S.; de Souza, R.C.A. COVID-19 and Digestive Endoscopy: Emergency Endoscopic Procedures and Risk Factors for Upper Gastrointestinal Bleeding. *Arq. Gastroenterol.* **2021**, *58*, 337–343. [CrossRef]
35. Zellmer, S.; Hanses, F.; Muzalyova, A.; Classen, J.; Braun, G.; Piepel, C.; Erber, J.; Pilgram, L.; Walter, L.; Göpel, S.; et al. Gastrointestinal bleeding and endoscopic findings in critically and non-critically ill patients with corona virus disease 2019 (COVID-19): Results from Lean European Open Survey on SARS-CoV-2 (LEOSS) and COKA registries. *United Eur. Gastroenterol. J.* **2021**, *9*, 1081–1090. [CrossRef] [PubMed]
36. Abowali, H.; Pacifico, A.; Erdinc, B.; Elkholy, K.; Burkhanova, U.; Aroriode, T.; Watson, A.; Ahmed, M.F.; Uwagbale, E.; Visweshwar, N.; et al. Assessment of Bleeding Risk in Hospitalized COVID-19 Patients: A Tertiary Hospital Experience during the Pandemic in a Predominant Minority Population—Bleeding Risk Factors in COVID-19 Patients. *J. Clin. Med.* **2022**, *11*, 2754. [CrossRef]
37. Abulawi, A.; Al-Tarbsheh, A.; Leamon, A.; Feustel, P.; Chopra, A.; Batool, A. Clinical Characteristics of Hospitalized COVID-19 Patients Who Have Gastrointestinal Bleeds Requiring Intervention: A Case-Control Study. *Cureus* **2022**, *14*, e26538. [CrossRef]
38. Shalimar; Vaishnav, M.; Elhence, A.; Kumar, R.; Mohta, S.; Palle, C.; Kumar, P.; Ranjan, M.; Vajpai, T.; Prasad, S.; et al. Outcome of Conservative Therapy in Coronavirus disease-2019 Patients Presenting With Gastrointestinal Bleeding. *J. Clin. Exp. Hepatol.* **2021**, *11*, 327–333. [CrossRef]
39. Lin, L.; Jiang, X.; Zhang, Z.; Huang, S.; Zhang, Z.; Fang, Z.; Gu, Z.; Gao, L.; Shi, H.; Mai, L.; et al. Gastrointestinal symptoms of 95 cases with SARS-CoV-2 infection. *Gut* **2020**, *69*, 997–1001. [CrossRef]
40. Shao, L.; Li, X.; Zhou, Y.; Yu, Y.; Liu, Y.; Liu, M.; Zhang, R.; Zhang, H.; Wang, X.; Zhou, F. Novel Insights into Illness Progression and Risk Profiles for Mortality in Non-survivors of COVID-19. *Front. Med.* **2020**, *7*, 246. [CrossRef]
41. Fanning, J.P.; Weaver, N.; Fanning, R.B.; Griffee, M.J.; Cho, S.-M.; Panigada, M.; Obonyo, N.G.; Zaaqoq, A.M.; Rando, H.; Chia, Y.W.; et al. Hemorrhage, Disseminated Intravascular Coagulopathy, and Thrombosis Complications Among Critically Ill Patients with COVID-19: An International COVID-19 Critical Care Consortium Study. *Crit. Care Med.* **2023**, *51*, 619–631. [CrossRef]
42. Zhao, X.; Tao, M.; Chen, C.; Zhang, Y.; Fu, Y. Clinical Features and Factors Associated with Occult Gastrointestinal Bleeding in COVID-19 Patients. *Infect. Drug Resist.* **2021**, *14*, 4217–4226. [CrossRef] [PubMed]
43. Martin, T.A.; Wan, D.W.; Hajifathalian, K.; Tewani, S.; Shah, S.L.; Mehta, A.; Kaplan, A.; Ghosh, G.; Choi, A.J.; Krisko, T.I.; et al. Gastrointestinal Bleeding in Patients with Coronavirus Disease 2019: A Matched Case-Control Study. *Am. J. Gastroenterol.* **2020**, *115*, 1609–1616. [CrossRef]
44. Xiao, F.; Tang, M.; Zheng, X.; Liu, Y.; Li, X.; Shan, H. Evidence for Gastrointestinal Infection of SARS-CoV-2. *Gastroenterology* **2020**, *158*, 1831–1833.e3. [CrossRef]
45. Al-Samkari, H.; Leaf, R.S.K.; Dzik, W.H.; Carlson, J.C.T.; Fogerty, A.E.; Waheed, A.; Goodarzi, K.; Bendapudi, P.K.; Bornikova, L.; Gupta, S.; et al. COVID-19 and coagulation: Bleeding and thrombotic manifestations of SARS-CoV-2 infection. *Blood* **2020**, *136*, 489–500. [CrossRef]
46. Wan, Y.; Li, J.; Shen, L.; Zou, Y.; Hou, L.; Zhu, L.; Faden, H.S.; Tang, Z.; Shi, M.; Jiao, N.; et al. Enteric involvement in hospitalised patients with COVID-19 outside Wuhan. *Lancet Gastroenterol. Hepatol.* **2020**, *5*, 534–535. [CrossRef] [PubMed]
47. Mattioli, M.; Benfaremo, D.; Mancini, M.; Mucci, L.; Mainquà, P.; Polenta, A.; Baldini, P.M.; Fulgenzi, F.; Dennetta, D.; Bedetta, S.; et al. Safety of intermediate dose of low molecular weight heparin in COVID-19 patients. *J. Thromb. Thrombolysis* **2021**, *51*, 286–292. [CrossRef] [PubMed]
48. Patell, R.; Bogue, T.; Bindal, P.; Koshy, A.; Merrill, M.; Aird, W.C.; Bauer, K.A.; Zwicker, J.I. Incidence of thrombosis and hemorrhage in hospitalized cancer patients with COVID-19. *J. Thromb. Haemost.* **2020**, *18*, 2349–2357. [CrossRef]
49. Bunch, C.M.; Thomas, A.V.; Stillson, J.E.; Gillespie, L.; Khan, R.Z.; Zackariya, N.; Shariff, F.; Al-Fadhl, M.; Mjaess, N.; Miller, P.D.; et al. Preventing Thrombohemorrhagic Complications of Heparinized COVID-19 Patients Using Adjunctive Thromboelastography: A Retrospective Study. *J. Clin. Med.* **2021**, *10*, 3097. [CrossRef]
50. Qiu, C.; Li, T.; Wei, G.; Xu, J.; Yu, W.; Wu, Z.; Li, D.; He, Y.; Chen, T.; Zhang, J.; et al. Hemorrhage and venous thromboembolism in critically ill patients with COVID-19. *SAGE Open Med.* **2021**, *9*, 1–8. [CrossRef]
51. Russell, L.; Weihe, S.; Madsen, E.K.; Hvas, C.L.; Leistner, J.W.; Michelsen, J.; Brøchner, A.C.; Bastiansen, A.; Nielsen, F.M.; Meier, N.; et al. Thromboembolic and bleeding events in ICU patients with COVID-19: A nationwide, observational study. *Acta Anaesthesiol. Scand.* **2023**, *67*, 76–85. [CrossRef]

52. Bychinin, M.V.; Klypa, T.V.; Mandel, I.A.; Avdonin, P.V.; Korshunov, D.I. Thrombotic and hemorrhagic complications in patients with severe and extremely severe COVID-19. *Anesteziol. Reanimatol.* **2022**, *2*, 24–32. [CrossRef]
53. Bonaffini, P.A.; Franco, P.N.; Bonanomi, A.; Giaccherini, C.; Valle, C.; Marra, P.; Norsa, L.; Marchetti, M.; Falanga, A.; Sironi, S. Ischemic and hemorrhagic abdominal complications in COVID-19 patients: Experience from the first Italian wave. *Eur. J. Med. Res.* **2022**, *27*, 165. [CrossRef]
54. Abdelmohsen, M.A.; Alkandari, B.M.; Gupta, V.K.; Elsebaie, N. Gastrointestinal tract imaging findings in confirmed COVID-19 patients: A non-comparative observational study. *Egypt. J. Radiol. Nucl. Med.* **2021**, *52*, 52. [CrossRef]
55. Neuberger, M.; Jungbluth, A.; Irlbeck, M.; Streitparth, F.; Burian, M.; Kirchner, T.; Werner, J.; Rudelius, M.; Knösel, T. Duodenal tropism of SARS-CoV-2 and clinical findings in critically ill COVID-19 patients. *Infection* **2022**, *50*, 1111–1120. [CrossRef] [PubMed]
56. Butorin, N.N.; Tsukanov, V.V.; Asyayev, R.V.; Butorina, M.N.; Vasyutin, A.V.; Tonkikh, J.L. The frequency of ulcerative-erosive defects and ulcerative bleeding of the gastroduodenal zone in patients with coronavirus infection COVID-19. *Exp. Clin. Gastroenterol.* **2022**, 5–11. [CrossRef]
57. Demelo-Rodriguez, P.; Galeano-Valle, F.; Ordieres-Ortega, L.; Siniscalchi, C.; Del Pozo, M.M.; Fidalgo, Á.; Gil-Díaz, A.; Lobo, J.L.; De Ancos, C.; Monreal, M.; et al. Validation of a Prognostic Score to Identify Hospitalized Patients with COVID-19 at Increased Risk for Bleeding. *Viruses* **2021**, *13*, 2278. [CrossRef]
58. Kalra, P.R.; Greenlaw, N.; Ferrari, R.; Ford, I.; Tardif, J.C.; Tendera, M.; Reid, C.M.; Danchin, N.; Stepinska, J.; Steg, P.G.; et al. Hemoglobin and Change in Hemoglobin Status Predict Mortality, Cardiovascular Events, and Bleeding in Stable Coronary Artery Disease. *Am. J. Med.* **2017**, *130*, 720–730. [CrossRef]
59. Barcellona, D.; Fenu, L.; Marongiu, F. Point-of-care testing INR: An overview. *Clin. Chem. Lab. Med. CCLM* **2017**, *55*, 800–805. [CrossRef]
60. Yang, R.; Moosavi, L. *Prothrombin Time*; StatPearls Publishing: Treasure Island, FL, USA, 2023.
61. Weitz, J.I.; Fredenburgh, J.C.; Eikelboom, J.W. A Test in Context: D-Dimer. *J. Am. Coll. Cardiol.* **2017**, *70*, 2411–2420. [CrossRef]
62. Kim, J.S.; Lee, J.Y.; Yang, J.W.; Lee, K.H.; Effenberger, M.; Szpirt, W.; Kronbichler, A.; Shin, J.I. Immunopathogenesis and treatment of cytokine storm in COVID-19. *Theranostics* **2021**, *11*, 316–329. [CrossRef]
63. Wagner, C.; Griesel, M.; Mikolajewska, A.; Mueller, A.; Nothacker, M.; Kley, K.; Metzendorf, M.-I.; Fischer, A.-L.; Kopp, M.; Stegemann, M.; et al. Systemic corticosteroids for the treatment of COVID-19. *Cochrane Database Syst. Rev.* **2021**, *2021*, CD014963. [CrossRef]
64. Chaudhuri, D.; Sasaki, K.; Karkar, A.; Sharif, S.; Lewis, K.; Mammen, M.J.; Alexander, P.; Ye, Z.; Lozano, L.E.C.; Munch, M.W.; et al. Corticosteroids in COVID-19 and non-COVID-19 ARDS: A systematic review and meta-analysis. *Intensive Care Med.* **2021**, *47*, 521–537. [CrossRef]
65. Halpin, D.M.G.; Singh, D.; Hadfield, R.M. Inhaled corticosteroids and COVID-19: A systematic review and clinical perspective. *Eur. Respir. J.* **2020**, *55*, 2001009. [CrossRef] [PubMed]
66. Xu, Y.; Siegal, D.M. Anticoagulant-associated gastrointestinal bleeding: Framework for decisions about whether, when and how to resume anticoagulants. *J. Thromb. Haemost.* **2021**, *19*, 2383–2393. [CrossRef] [PubMed]
67. Barnes, G.D.; Burnett, A.; Allen, A.; Ansell, J.; Blumenstein, M.; Clark, N.P.; Crowther, M.; Dager, W.E.; Deitelzweig, S.B.; Ellsworth, S.; et al. Thromboembolic prevention and anticoagulant therapy during the COVID-19 pandemic: Updated clinical guidance from the anticoagulation forum. *J. Thromb. Thrombolysis* **2022**, *54*, 197–210. [CrossRef] [PubMed]
68. Asakura, H.; Ogawa, H. COVID-19-associated coagulopathy and disseminated intravascular coagulation. *Int. J. Hematol.* **2021**, *113*, 45–57. [CrossRef]
69. Gómez-Mesa, J.E.; Galindo-Coral, S.; Montes, M.C.; Martin, A.J.M. Thrombosis and Coagulopathy in COVID-19. *Curr. Probl. Cardiol.* **2021**, *46*, 100742. [CrossRef]
70. Miesbach, W.; Makris, M. COVID-19: Coagulopathy, Risk of Thrombosis, and the Rationale for Anticoagulation. *Clin. Appl. Thromb. Hemost.* **2020**, *26*, 1–7. [CrossRef]
71. Iba, T.; Connors, J.M.; Levy, J.H. The coagulopathy, endotheliopathy, and vasculitis of COVID-19. *Inflamm. Res.* **2020**, *69*, 1181–1189. [CrossRef]
72. Kherad, O.; Restellini, S.; Martel, M.; Barkun, A. Proton pump inhibitors for upper gastrointestinal bleeding. *Best Pract. Res. Clin. Gastroenterol.* **2019**, *42–43*, 101609. [CrossRef] [PubMed]
73. Barkun, A.N.; Almadi, M.; Kuipers, E.J.; Laine, L.; Sung, J.; Tse, F.; Leontiadis, G.I.; Abraham, N.S.; Calvet, X.; Chan, F.K.; et al. Management of Nonvariceal Upper Gastrointestinal Bleeding: Guideline Recommendations from the International Consensus Group. *Ann. Intern. Med.* **2019**, *171*, 805. [CrossRef] [PubMed]
74. Laine, L.; Jensen, D.M. Management of Patients with Ulcer Bleeding. *Am. J. Gastroenterol.* **2012**, *107*, 345–360. [CrossRef] [PubMed]
75. Cavaliere, K.; Levine, C.; Wander, P.; Sejpal, D.V.; Trindade, A.J. Management of upper GI bleeding in patients with COVID-19 pneumonia. *Gastrointest. Endosc.* **2020**, *92*, 454–455. [CrossRef] [PubMed]
76. Patel, P.; Sengupta, N. PPIs and Beyond: A Framework for Managing Anticoagulation-Related Gastrointestinal Bleeding in the Era of COVID-19. *Dig. Dis. Sci.* **2020**, *65*, 2181–2186. [CrossRef] [PubMed]
77. Sauerbruch, T.; Fischer, G. Conservative treatment of upper gastrointestinal bleeding in portal hypertension. *Hepatogastroenterology* **1991**, *38*, 350–354. [PubMed]

78. Gralnek, I.M.; Stanley, A.J.; Morris, A.J.; Camus, M.; Lau, J.; Lanas, A.; Laursen, S.B.; Radaelli, F.; Papanikolaou, I.S.; Gonçalves, T.C.; et al. Endoscopic diagnosis and management of nonvariceal upper gastrointestinal hemorrhage (NVUGIH): European Society of Gastrointestinal Endoscopy (ESGE) Guideline—Update 2021. *Endoscopy* **2021**, *53*, 300–332. [CrossRef]
79. Strate, L.L.; Gralnek, I.M. ACG Clinical Guideline: Management of Patients with Acute Lower Gastrointestinal Bleeding. *Am. J. Gastroenterol.* **2016**, *111*, 459–474. [CrossRef]
80. Nett, A.; Binmoeller, K.F. Endoscopic Management of Portal Hypertension–related Bleeding. *Gastrointest. Endosc. Clin. N. Am.* **2019**, *29*, 321–337. [CrossRef]
81. Bujanda, L.; Arratibel, P.; Gil, I.; Torrente, S.; Martos, M.; Enriquez-Navascues, J.M. Surgery and emergency gastrointestinal endoscopy during the Covid-19 pandemic. *Gastroenterol. Hepatol.* **2021**, *44*, 294–296. [CrossRef]
82. Benites-Goñi, H.; Pascacio-Fiori, M.; Valle, F.M.-D.; Plácido-Damián, Z.; Gonzales-Carazas, E.; Padilla-Espinoza, M.; Prado-Bustamante, J.; Llatas-Pérez, J.; Dávalos-Moscol, M. Impact of the COVID-19 pandemic in the time to endoscopy in patients with upper gastrointestinal bleedin. *Rev. Gastroenterol. Peru* **2020**, *40*, 219–223. [CrossRef] [PubMed]
83. Ierardi, A.M.; Coppola, A.; Tortora, S.; Valconi, E.; Piacentino, F.; Fontana, F.; Stellato, E.; Cogliati, C.B.; Torzillo, D.; Giampalma, E.; et al. Gastrointestinal Bleeding in Patients with SARS-CoV-2 Infection Managed by Interventional Radiology. *J. Clin. Med.* **2021**, *10*, 4758. [CrossRef]
84. Ierardi, A.M.; Del Giudice, C.; Coppola, A.; Carnevale, A.; Giganti, M.; Renzulli, M.; Tacher, V.; Urbano, J.; Kobeiter, H.; Loffroy, R.; et al. Gastrointestinal Hemorrhages in Patients With COVID-19 Managed With Transarterial Embolization. *Am. J. Gastroenterol.* **2021**, *116*, 838–840. [CrossRef]
85. Tavabie, O.D.; Clough, J.N.; Blackwell, J.; Bashyam, M.; Martin, H.; Soubieres, A.; Direkze, N.; Graham, D.; Groves, C.; Preston, S.L.; et al. Reduced survival after upper gastrointestinal bleed endoscopy in the COVID-19 era is a secondary effect of the response to the global pandemic: A retrospective cohort study. *Frontline Gastroenterol.* **2021**, *12*, 279–287. [CrossRef] [PubMed]
86. Barrett, L.F.; Lo, K.B.; Stanek, S.R.; Walter, J.W. Self-limited gastrointestinal bleeding in COVID-19. *Clin. Res. Hepatol. Gastroenterol.* **2020**, *44*, e77–e80. [CrossRef] [PubMed]
87. Blackett, J.W.; Kumta, N.A.; Dixon, R.E.; David, Y.; Nagula, S.; DiMaio, C.J.; Greenwald, D.; Sharaiha, R.Z.; Sampath, K.; Carr-Locke, D.; et al. Characteristics and Outcomes of Patients Undergoing Endoscopy during the COVID-19 Pandemic: A Multicenter Study from New York City. *Dig. Dis. Sci.* **2021**, *66*, 2545–2554. [CrossRef] [PubMed]
88. Adekunle, A.D.; Rubens, M.; Sedarous, M.; Tariq, T.; Okafor, P.N. Trends in gastrointestinal disease hospitalizations and outcomes during the first year of the coronavirus pandemic. *World J. Gastroenterol.* **2023**, *29*, 744–757. [CrossRef]
89. Rehana, R.W.; Fahad, H.; Sadiq, O.; Schairer, J. Outcomes of Gastrointestinal Bleeding During the COVID-19 Pandemic. *Gastro Hep Adv.* **2022**, *1*, 342–343. [CrossRef]
90. Iqbal, U.; Patel, P.D.; Pluskota, C.A.; Berger, A.L.; Khara, H.S.; Confer, B.D. Outcomes of Acute Gastrointestinal Bleeding in Patients With COVID-19: A Case-Control Study. *Gastroenterol. Res.* **2022**, *15*, 13–18. [CrossRef]
91. Reddy, S.; Patel, B.; Baldelli, L.; Majithia, R.T.; Dougherty, M.K. Decreased Rate of Presentation, but Worsened Racial-Ethnic Disparity in Acute Gastrointestinal Bleeding During Coronavirus 2019 Shutdown: A Retrospective Cohort Study. *Clin. Exp. Gastroenterol.* **2022**, *15*, 67–77. [CrossRef]
92. Smith, R.; Brooks, C.; Rammage, J. Short report on acute gastro-intestinal bleeding admissions during the COVID-19 pandemic. *JGH Open* **2022**, *6*, 263–265. [CrossRef] [PubMed]
93. Wilkins, T.; Wheeler, B.; Carpenter, M. Upper Gastrointestinal Bleeding in Adults: Evaluation and Management. *Am. Fam. Physician* **2020**, *101*, 294–300. [PubMed]
94. Samuel, R.; Bilal, M.; Tayyem, O.; Guturu, P. Evaluation and management of Non-variceal upper gastrointestinal bleeding. *Dis. A Mon.* **2018**, *64*, 333–343. [CrossRef] [PubMed]
95. García-Rayado, G.; Lanas, A. Upper gastrointestinal bleeding in critically ill patients: Proton-pump inhibitors, histamine-2 receptor antagonists or placebo? Many questions remain unanswered. *Curr. Med. Res. Opin.* **2018**, *34*, 1881–1883. [CrossRef] [PubMed]
96. Bardou, M.; Quenot, J.-P.; Barkun, A. Stress-related mucosal disease in the critically ill patient. *Nat. Rev. Gastroenterol. Hepatol.* **2015**, *12*, 98–107. [CrossRef] [PubMed]
97. Gupta, A.; Madhavan, M.V.; Sehgal, K.; Nair, N.; Mahajan, S.; Sehrawat, T.S.; Bikdeli, B.; Ahluwalia, N.; Ausiello, J.C.; Wan, E.Y.; et al. Extrapulmonary manifestations of COVID-19. *Nat. Med.* **2020**, *26*, 1017–1032. [CrossRef] [PubMed]
98. Abu-Ssaydeh, D.A.; Rechnitzer, T.W.; Knowles, B.P.; Richmond, T.S. Major haemorrhage associated with the Flexi-Seal® Fecal Management System. *Anaesth. Intensive Care* **2018**, *46*, 140. [PubMed]
99. Tiwari, A.; Sharma, H.; Qamar, K.; Alastal, Y.; Sodeman, T.; Nawras, A. The Traumatic Tube: Bleeding Rectal Ulcer Caused by Flexi-Seal Device. *Case Rep. Gastrointest Med.* **2017**, *2017*, 5278971. [CrossRef]
100. Padmanabhan, A.; Stern, M.; Wishin, J.; Mangino, M.; Richey, K.; DeSane, M.; Flexi-Seal Clinical Trial Investigators Group. Clinical evaluation of a flexible fecal incontinence management system. *Am. J. Crit. Care* **2007**, *16*, 384–393. [CrossRef]
101. Akinosoglou, K.; Savopoulos, C.; Pouliakis, A.; Triantafyllidis, C.; Markatis, E.; Golemi, F.; Liontos, A.; Vadala, C.; Papanikolaou, I.C.; Dimakopoulou, V.; et al. Intensive-Dose Tinzaparin in Hospitalized COVID-19 Patients: The INTERACT Study. *Viruses* **2022**, *14*, 767. [CrossRef]
102. Goligher, E.C.; Bradbury, C.A.; McVerry, B.J.; Lawler, P.R.; Berger, J.S.; Gong, M.N. Therapeutic Anticoagulation with Heparin in Critically Ill Patients with Covid-19. *N. Engl. J. Med.* **2021**, *385*, 777–789. [CrossRef]

103. Cate, H.T. Surviving Covid-19 with Heparin? *N. Engl. J. Med.* **2021**, *385*, 845–846. [CrossRef]
104. Leung, W.K.; To, K.-F.; Chan, P.K.; Chan, H.L.; Wu, A.K.; Lee, N.; Yuen, K.Y.; Sung, J.J. Enteric involvement of severe acute respiratory syndrome-associated coronavirus infection. *Gastroenterology* **2003**, *125*, 1011–1017. [CrossRef]
105. Marasco, G.; Maida, M.; Morreale, G.C.; Licata, M.; Renzulli, M.; Cremon, C.; Stanghellini, V.; Barbara, G. Gastrointestinal Bleeding in COVID-19 Patients: A Systematic Review with Meta-Analysis. *Can. J. Gastroenterol. Hepatol.* **2021**, *2021*, 2534975. [CrossRef]

Disclaimer/Publisher's Note: The statements, opinions and data contained in all publications are solely those of the individual author(s) and contributor(s) and not of MDPI and/or the editor(s). MDPI and/or the editor(s) disclaim responsibility for any injury to people or property resulting from any ideas, methods, instructions or products referred to in the content.

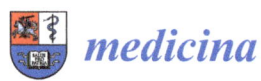

Brief Report

Antibody Kinetics after Three Doses of SARS-CoV-2 mRNA Vaccination in Patients with Inflammatory Bowel Disease

Evangelos Tsipotis [1], Ankith Maremanda [2], Laura Bowles Zeiser [3], Caoilfhionn Connolly [4], Sowmya Sharma [2], Sharon Dudley-Brown [2], Sarah Frey [5], Mark Lazarev [2], Joanna M. Melia [2], Alyssa M. Parian [2], Dorry L. Segev [6], Brindusa Truta [2], Huimin Yu [2], William A. Werbel [7,*] and Florin M. Selaru [2,8,*]

[1] Digestive Health Center, Augusta University, Augusta, GA 30912, USA; v.tsipotis@yahoo.com
[2] Hopkins IBD Center, Division of Gastroenterology, Department of Medicine, Johns Hopkins University School of Medicine, Baltimore, MD 21224, USA; amarema1@jhu.edu (A.M.); ssharm85@jh.edu (S.S.); sdudley2@jhmi.edu (S.D.-B.); mlazare1@jhmi.edu (M.L.); joanna.peloquin@jhmi.edu (J.M.M.); aparian1@jhmi.edu (A.M.P.); btruta1@jhmi.edu (B.T.); hyu20@jhmi.edu (H.Y.)
[3] Department of Surgery, NYU Grossman School of Medicine, New York, NY 10016, USA; laura.zeiser@nyulangone.org
[4] Division of Rheumatology, Department of Medicine, Johns Hopkins University School of Medicine, Baltimore, MD 21224, USA; cconno15@jhmi.edu
[5] Department of Surgery, Johns Hopkins University School of Medicine, Baltimore, MD 21224, USA; sfrey6@jhmi.edu
[6] Department of Surgery Center for Surgical and Transplant Applied Research, NYU Langone Health, New York, NY 10016, USA; dorry@jhmi.edu
[7] Division of Infectious Diseases, Department of Medicine, Johns Hopkins University School of Medicine, Baltimore, MD 21224, USA
[8] Sidney Kimmel Comprehensive Cancer Center, Johns Hopkins University, Baltimore, MD 21224, USA
* Correspondence: wwerbel1@jhmi.edu (W.A.W.); fselaru1@jhmi.edu (F.M.S.); Tel.: +1-410-614-3801 (F.M.S.)

Abstract: *Background:* The emergence of new SARS-CoV-2 variants calls for more data on SARS-CoV-2 mRNA vaccine response. *Aims:* We aimed to assess the response to a third mRNA vaccine dose against SARS-CoV-2 in inflammatory bowel disease (IBD) patients. *Methods:* This was a single-center, observational prospective study of IBD patients who received a third mRNA vaccine dose against SARS-CoV-2. Antibody titers were taken post-third-dose at one and three months using the Roche Elecsys anti-SARS-CoV-2-S enzyme immunoassay. Titers less than 0.8 units/mL were considered negative according to the manufactures. Titers between 0.8 units/mL and 250 units/mL were considered non-neutralizing. Titers greater than 250 units/mL were considered neutralizing. *Results:* Eighty-three patients were included, all of whom had detectable antibodies at 3 months post-third dose. A total of 89% showed neutralizing and 11% non-neutralizing titers. Participants with non-neutralizing titers were more likely to be on systemic corticosteroids ($p = 0.04$). Two participants seroconverted from negative to positive, whereas 86% with non-neutralizing titers boosted to neutralizing levels. Only one participant with neutralizing titers after a third dose had a decrease to a non-neutralizing level within 3 months. *Conclusions:* Our findings support the ongoing recommendations for additional doses in immunocompromised individuals. However, longitudinal studies with a greater-sized patient population are needed.

Keywords: COVID-19; SARS-CoV-2; vaccination; IBD

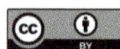

1. Introduction

Initial findings have demonstrated that the majority of patients with inflammatory bowel disease (IBD), including those with Ulcerative Colitis (UC) and/or Crohn's Disease (CD), develop antibodies that persist for at least 6 months following a two-dose series of SARS-CoV-2 mRNA vaccines [1–3]. However, an attenuated antibody response (a lower concentration of anti-SARS-CoV-2 antibodies) has been observed in individuals who are taking corticosteroids, Tumor Necrosis Factor (TNF-a) inhibitors, or combination therapies (the concurrent use of biologic medications and immunosuppressive treatments, which may include thiopurines like 6-mercaptopurine and azathioprine, as well as corticosteroids) [4–6]. These therapies are important for the management of IBD, and oftentimes, the magnitude of disease activity necessitates the continuation of these therapies regardless of vaccine prophylaxis of SARS-CoV-2. Consequently, the diminished antibody response following vaccination in these patients is concerning.

Moreover, subsequent to those studies, the emergence of the SARS-CoV-2 Omicron variant (BA.1/B.1.1.529) and its sublineages, which exhibit significant immune evasion and transmissibility, has been observed. The Omicron variant, identified in Africa in November 2021, possesses up to 32 mutations in the receptor-binding domain (RBD) and N-terminal domain of the spike protein, in comparison to the original variant. As the spike protein is the target of neutralizing antibodies, the presence of these mutations may enhance the virus's ability to evade antibodies, thereby contributing to an increased viral fitness [7]. Recent studies have indicated that achieving neutralization in immunocompromised patients might require higher antibody titers [8,9].

In an effort to address waning antibody responses and enhance protection against novel SARS-CoV-2 variants such as Omicron and Delta (B.1.617.2) pseudo viruses, among others, the Advisory Committee on Immunization Practices (ACIP) of the Centers for Disease Control and Prevention (CDC) has recommended a third primary mRNA vaccine dose for individuals with moderate-to-severe immunocompromization. Additionally, booster doses are recommended for all individuals aged 5 years and above, at least four months after completing the initial mRNA vaccine series [10].

Initial studies in IBD patients show that the third dose may be safe to administer. A single-center study by Pellegrino et al. showed no repercussions in IBD patients to whom the BNT162b2 vaccine (Pfizer-BioNTech) was administered [11]. Additionally, Li et al.'s study showed that symptoms for IBD patients after a third mRNA vaccine dose tended to be milder than symptoms manifested after the second dose [12].

We conducted a single-center, observational prospective study to investigate 1-month and 3-month outcomes in IBD patients who received their third mRNA vaccine doses.

2. Materials and Methods
2.1. Patient Recruitment

Our study included English-speaking adult patients, defined as 18 years and older, who are living in the United States and have been diagnosed with IBD. These patients are maintained on immunosuppression treatment for IBD and/or have other coexisting conditions with an immune-mediated etiology. Additionally, they received three doses of FDA-approved mRNA vaccines (mRNA-1273 manufactured by Moderna or BNT162b2 manufactured by Pfizer-BioNTech). Those who had a prior COVID-19 infection were eligible to participate in the study. To track baseline demographics (age, sex, race) and clinical notes, including a list of medications patients were taking at the time of the study (including both IBD and non-IBD meds), we utilized a secure online form on a website maintained by the study team. Patients who received the third vaccine dose but had no prior information about their titer levels pre-third dose were not eligible for the study. Additionally, patients who did not speak English were excluded due to the lack of IRB approval for non-English consenting scripts. This study was approved by the Johns Hopkins Institutional Review Board (IRB00248540). Participants were notified about the study through alerts on their health portals (EPIC Systems Corporation) and by their physicians. They were informed that the study does not provide the vaccine, and study team members will not offer any guidance regarding whether one should receive the booster. Confirmation of the receipt of the third dose was obtained through communication with the patient and chart review. Informed consent was explicitly obtained from all participants before their inclusion in the study.

2.2. Titer Measurements

Antibody titers were measured using the Roche Elecsys anti-SARS-CoV-2-S enzyme immunoassay (EIA), which is a pan-immunoglobulin assay targeting the spike protein RBD. Titer measurements were performed at local clinical laboratories in Baltimore, Maryland, USA (Laboratory Corporation of America Holdings-LabCorp, Burlington, NC, USA). Measurements were taken before administration of the third mRNA vaccine dose, as well as one and three months after administration of the third dose. Titers less than 0.8 units/mL were considered negative according to manufacturer guidelines, and the assay's saturation limit was 2500 units/mL. Based on live virus-neutralizing antibody data in immunosuppressed populations, titers ranging from 0.8 to 250 units/mL were considered non-neutralizing, while titers greater than 250 units/mL were considered neutralizing [7,8].

2.3. Software Used

Data analysis was conducted using STATA software version 17.0 (StataCorp, College Station, TX, USA). Study data, including baseline demographics and medication records, were collected and managed using REDCap secure electronic data capture tools (version 11.0.3) hosted at Johns Hopkins University (Baltimore, MD, USA). Tables were generated using Microsoft Word.

3. Results

In our study, 83 IBD patients completed a three-dose SARS-CoV-2 mRNA vaccination regimen and had paired antibody testing performed prior to the administration of the third dose and at one and three months following the third vaccination dose (Tables 1 and 2). The median age of participants was 45.2 years, with a female predominance (72.2%). A total of 28.9% of patients in the study had an additional co-existing diagnosis of rheumatic disease (RMD).

The majority of patients (57.8%) received mRNA1273 (Moderna, Cambridge, MA, USA) as their third dose, with a mean (SD) interval of 154 (46.9) days from the second dose. The remaining 42.2% received BNT162b2 (Pfizer-BioNTech, Mainz, Germany) with a mean (SD) interval of 172 (39.8) days after the second dose. These findings indicate that most patients did not receive the third dose within one month after the administration of the second dose, as recommended by the CDC for individuals with moderate-to-severe immunocompromization (See Table 1 for details).

Among those who had non-neutralizing antibody levels, the majority were vaccinated with Moderna (five participants, 55.6%) and the mean (SD) time from second to third dose was 154 (46.9) days (Table 1). In this antibody titer group, five (55.6%) were being treated with anti-TNF-a inhibitors and one participant (11.1%) was on combination therapy of a systemic steroid with anti-TNF-a. Two participants (22.2%) were on mycophenolate mofetil.

Amongst the 83 participants, 1 participant (11.1%) with low titers had a flare post-vaccination with a third dose. No other adverse events were reported amongst our participants.

All participants with titers available at 3 months post-third dose had antibody titers checked before receiving the third dose. Table 2 summarizes the kinetics of antibody titers before and after the third dose. Prior to a third dose, 82 (98.8%) participants had detectable antibodies, including 42 (50.6%) with non-neutralizing titers, and only 2 (2.4%) had negative titers before the third dose. One patient was on infliximab monotherapy, and the other patient was on steroids, mycophenolate mofetil, and tacrolimus. Both patients developed positive but non-neutralizing antibody levels after the third dose.

At both 1 and 3 months post-third dose, 100% of participants had detectable antibodies, of whom 74 (89.2%) showed neutralizing titers and 9 (10.8%) showed non-neutralizing titers at 3 months (Table 2). Notably, the two participants who seroconverted from negative to positive after a third vaccine dose demonstrated non-neutralizing titers at 3 months, whereas 36 out of 42 participants (86%) with non-neutralizing titers boosted to neutralizing levels. Only 1 out of 40 participants (2.5%) attaining neutralizing titers after a third vaccine dose demonstrated a wane to non-neutralizing level by 3 months.

Table 1. Demographic and clinical characteristics of IBD patients after the administration of three-dose SARS-CoV-2 mRNA vaccination regimen.

	Non-Neutralizing Antibody Levels (n = 9) [1]	Neutralizing Antibody Levels (n = 74) [1]
Age, mean (SD)	50.3 (13.2)	47.2 (13.4)
Age, median (MAD)	44.8 (10.0)	45.2 (10.2)
Female sex, no. (%)	5 (55.6)	55 (74.3)
Non-white, no. (%)	0	4 (5.4)
RMD diagnosis, no. (%) [2]		
Lupus	0	0
Arthritis	2 (22.2)	14 (18.9)
Sjogrens	1 (11.1)	1 (1.4)
Myositis	2 (22.2)	1 (1.4)
Scleroderma	1 (11.1)	0
Vasculitis	1 (11.1)	0
Other	0	1 (1.4)
Total	7 (77.8)	17 (23.0)
Non-Biologics		
Meds used in IBD, no. (%)		
5-ASA [3]	0	2 (2.7)
Thiopurine [4]	0	14 (18.9)
Methotrexate	1 (11.1)	1 (1.4)
Tofacitinib	0	2 (2.7)
Non-IBD meds, no. (%)		
Hydroxychloroquine [5]	0	3 (4.0)
Mycophenolate [6]	2 (22.2)	2 (2.7)
Tacrolimus	1 (11.1)	1 (1.4)
Cyclosporine	0	1 (1.4)
Leflunomide	0	1 (1.4)
Biologics		
TNF inhibitor [7]	5 (55.6)	37 (50.0)
TNF inhibitor monotherapy	4 (44.4)	26 (35.1)
Ustekinumab	0	16 (21.6)
Vedolizumab	0	1 (1.4)
Etanercept	0	1 (1.4)
Corticosteroids		
Budesonide	0	4 (5.4)
Systemic Corticosteroid [8]	5 (55.6)	8 (10.8) *
Combination therapy		
TNF inhibitor [7] and thiopurine [4] or methotrexate	0	7 (9.4)
TNF inhibitor [7] and corticosteroid [8]	1 (11.1)	2 (2.7)
Medication held before vaccine, no. (%)		
Yes	4 (44.4)	10 (13.5) *
Vaccine, no (%)		
BNT162b2	4 (44.4)	31 (41.9)
mRNA-1273	5 (55.6)	43 (58.1)
Time from second to third dose (SD)	146 (30.5)	172 (40.1)
Mean (SD) anti-RBD	115.2 (68.8)	1980.4 (756.9)
Flare, no. (%)	1 (11.1)	3 (4.0)

SD (Standard Deviation), MAD (Median Absolute Deviation), RMD (Rheumatic and Musculoskeletal Diseases), 5-ASA (5-aminosalicylic acid), TNF (Tumor Necrosis Factor). [1] Percentages in the columns are represented as percent of each category in the overall column. Negative antibody response was defined as Roche Elecsys anti-RBD pan Ig less than 0.8 u/mL. Non-neutralizing antibody titers were defined as anti-RBD pan Ig 0.8 to 250 u/mL. Neutralizing antibody titers defined as anti-RBD pan Ig greater than or equal to 250 u/mL. No participant had negative antibody titers at 3 months post-vaccination with a third dose. [2] Participants also have a diagnosis of systemic lupus erythematosus, myositis, Sjögren's syndrome, rheumatoid arthritis, systemic sclerosis, ankylosing spondylitis, reactive arthritis, inflammatory bowel disease associated arthritis, psoriatic arthritis, polyarteritis nodosa, polymyalgia rheumatica, temporal arteritis, Behcet's syndrome, eosinophilic granulomatosis polyangiitis, Henoch–Schonlein purpura, granulomatous polyangiitis, Takayasu's arteritis, or microscopic polyangiitis. [3] 5-ASA includes prescription of mesalamine, sulfasalazine, and olsalazine. [4] Thiopurines include prescription of azathioprine and 6-mercaptopurine (6-MP). [5] Hydroxychloroquine includes prescription of hydroxychloroquine and chloroquine. [6] Mycophenolate includes prescription of mycophenolate mofetil and mycophenolic acid. [7] TNF-a inhibitors include prescription of adalimumab, infliximab, certolizumab-pegol, golimumab, and etanercept. [8] Other corticosteroid includes prescription of prednisone and prednisone equivalents (such as prednisolone). * Indicates that the two groups were statistically significantly different using Fisher exact test. p-value for systemic cosrticosteroids was 0.004 and for holding medication was 0.038.

Table 2. Antibody response against SARS-CoV-2 spike protein three months following two doses of SARS-CoV-2 vaccine in patients with IBD, stratified by a one-month antibody response after mRNA three-dose series.

		Antibodies Three Months after D3			
		Negative	Non-neutralizing titers	Neutralizing titers	Total
Antibodies-before D3	Negative	0	2	0	2
	Non-neutralizing titers	0	6	36	42
	Neutralizing titers	0	1	38	39
	Total	0	9	74	83

Negative response was defined as Roche Elecsys anti-RBD pan Ig less than 0.8 u/mL. Non-neutralizing antibody titers were defined as anti-RBD pan Ig 0.8 to 250 u/mL. Neutralizing antibody titers were defined as anti-RBD pan Ig greater than or equal to 250 u/mL. A total of 74 participants (89.2%) exhibited neutralizing antibody titers, while 9 participants (10.8%) showed positive but non-neutralizing antibody titers at three months following administration of a third vaccine dose. Among those with neutralizing antibody levels, the most commonly prescribed medication was TNF-a inhibitors, which were being used by 37 patients (50.0%). Treatment with thiopurines was observed in only 14 patients (18.9%), corticosteroids in 8 patients (10.8%), and budesonide in 4 patients (5.4%). Additionally, 7 participants (9.5%) with neutralizing antibody levels were receiving a combination of anti-TNF-a therapy with thiopurines or methotrexate, and 2 participants (2.7%) were on a combination of an anti-TNF-a medication with systemic corticosteroids. Three patients (3.6%) with high antibody titers experienced a flare-up following vaccination.

In contrasting antibody response groups, baseline characteristics were similar, as was the use of TNFa inhibitor therapy. Participants with non-neutralizing titers, however, were more likely to be taking systemic corticosteroid therapy (5/9 vs. 8/74, $p = 0.04$) and have peri-vaccination immunosuppressive held (4/9 vs. 10/74, $p = 0.038$). IBD flares were reported in one (11.1%) of the non-neutralizing titer group and three (4%) of the neutralizing titer group.

4. Discussion

In this study, we observed a neutralizing anti-RBD antibody titer response in the majority of IBD patients (89.2%) who received a third dose of an FDA-approved SARS-CoV-2 mRNA vaccine at least 3 months post-vaccination, using the currently recommended definition of high antibody titers. None of the participants had negative titers after receiving the third dose. Two participants had negative titers before the third dose but developed antibodies after receiving the vaccine. Only one participant (2.5%) with neutralizing titers before the third dose experienced a decrease to non-neutralizing titers at 3 months after vaccination. Two patients (2.4%) had non-neutralizing titers prior to the booster dose, and their titers remained non-neutralizing even after vaccination. These patients were either on infliximab or a combination of mycophenolate mofetil and tacrolimus. Among the four participants (4.8%) who experienced a flare, three had neutralizing titers. It is currently unclear why the majority of patients who flared were in the neutralizing titer group. One possible explanation could be that, compared to the low titer group, a lower proportion of patients in the high titer group were on anti-TNF-a therapy or systemic corticosteroids, indicating a possible poor control of their disease. Unfortunately, we did not have any data regarding the disease severity and activity among the groups. Interestingly, participants with non-neutralizing titers were more likely to be taking systemic corticosteroid therapy. Although there is limited existing literature on this topic, one systematic review showed that risk factors for not responding to SARS-CoV-2 vaccination included systemic corticosteroid usage [13].

Other studies have reported similar outcomes to ours. A multicenter prospective study involving the University of Wisconsin-Madison (Madison, WI, USA) and Mayo Clinic (Jacksonville, FL, USA) demonstrated that all IBD patients who received a third SARS-CoV-2 mRNA vaccine dose exhibited a humoral immune response [14]. Additionally, another study showed that IBD patients on similar treatment regimens to those in our study were able to mount a serological response comparable to a control group following the administration of a third dose [15]. A study focusing on patients with autoinflammatory rheumatic and musculoskeletal diseases also showed an increased humoral response in the majority of participants following the administration of a third SARS-CoV-2 mRNA vaccine dose [16].

Preventative health screening, including updated vaccinations for vaccine-preventable diseases, is a crucial aspect of IBD patient management. Providers who care for the IBD community must address the concerns and hesitations surrounding the SARS-CoV-2 vaccine. One study aimed at assessing the sentiments of IBD patients regarding the vaccine found that 33% of those surveyed were hesitant to get vaccinated primarily due to concerns about vaccine safety and efficacy [17]. We demonstrated that the administration of a third mRNA vaccine dose resulted in a neutralizing response in the majority of IBD patients, confirming the efficacy of the vaccine. Our results align with numerous other studies examining IBD patients receiving a third SARS-CoV-2 mRNA vaccine, providing consistent evidence of a humoral immune response. We hope that this can contribute to increasing confidence in SARS-CoV-2 vaccination for populations with IBD.

Some limitations of our study include a small sample size and a lack of racial and ethnic diversity within our patient population, with the majority of participants being white.

Furthermore, this study is limited by the absence of formal neutralization testing against variants of concern and the lack of anti-nucleocapsid testing to monitor subclinical infections or prior exposure. Additionally, the exact vaccine doses administered were not ascertainable. No testing was conducted to exclude breakthrough infections that could have resulted in sustained antibody titers in some participants. Longitudinal studies that include a diverse representation of IBD patients across the spectrum of disease activity are necessary to comprehensively assess the depth and durability of immune responses in this complex group with varying phenotypes.

Ultimately, our findings are consistent with other studies that have examined anti-RBD kinetics after both two and three doses of mRNA vaccination in IBD patients, as well as patients with other autoinflammatory diseases. These studies demonstrate that mRNA vaccines are safe for use in the IBD population [5,14–16].

5. Conclusions

In conclusion, the results of our study support the ongoing recommendation of the CDC for additional doses of SARS-CoV-2 mRNA vaccines in immunocompromised patients. While these initial results are encouraging and provide insight into the responsiveness of patients with IBD to a third mRNA vaccine dose, more comprehensive research involving a larger patient population and a longer time span is needed.

Author Contributions: E.T., Study conceptualization and design, acquisition of data, interpretation of data, drafting of the manuscript, critical revision of the manuscript for important intellectual content; A.M., study conceptualization and design, acquisition of data, analysis and interpretation of data, drafting of the manuscript, critical revision of the manuscript for important intellectual content; L.B.Z., acquisition of data, review and editing of manuscript; S.F., review and editing of manuscript; C.C., study conceptualization and design, interpretation of data, drafting of the manuscript, critical revision of the manuscript for important intellectual content; S.S., reviewing and editing of the manuscript; S.D.-B., review and editing of manuscript; M.L., review and editing of manuscript; J.M.M., review and editing of manuscript; A.M.P., review and editing of manuscript; B.T., review and editing of manuscript; H.Y., review and editing of manuscript; D.L.S., study conceptualization, interpretation of data, drafting of the manuscript, critical revision of the manuscript for important intellectual content, study supervision, funding acquisition; W.A.W., study conceptualization and design, interpretation of data, drafting of the manuscript, critical revision of the manuscript for important intellectual content; F.M.S., study conceptualization and design, interpretation of data, drafting of the manuscript, critical revision of the manuscript for important intellectual content. All authors have read and agreed to the published version of the manuscript.

Funding: This work was made possible by the generous support of the Ben-Dov and Trokhan Patterson families. This work was supported by the Jerome L. Greene Foundation Discovery Fund (Connolly) and grant number T32DK007713 (Alejo) from the National Institute of Diabetes and

Digestive and Kidney Diseases (NIDDK), K24AI144954 (Segev), U01AI138897-S04 and K23AI157893 (Werbel) from National Institute of Allergy and Infectious Diseases (NIAID). The analyses described here are the responsibility of the authors alone and do not necessarily reflect the views or policies of the Department of Health and Human Services, nor do the mentioned trade names, commercial products, or organizations imply endorsement by the US Government.

Institutional Review Board Statement: The study was conducted according to the guidelines of the Declaration of Helsinki, and approved by the Institutional Review Board (or Ethics Committee) of Johns Hopkins University (IRB00248540 and 8 May 2022).

Informed Consent Statement: Informed consent was obtained from all subjects involved in the study.

Data Availability Statement: The data underlying this article will be shared on reasonable request to the corresponding author.

Acknowledgments: The authors thank the participants of our study, without whom this work would have been impossible, as well as the Johns Hopkins transplant vaccine study team, including Brian Boyarsky, Jennifer Alejo, Mayan Teles, and Teresa Po-Yu Chiang.

Conflicts of Interest: Segev reports receiving honoraria from Sanofi (speaking), Novartis (speaking, consulting), Veloxis (consulting), Mallinckrodt (consulting), Jazz Pharmaceuticals (consulting), CSL Behring (consulting), Thermo Fisher Scientific (consulting), Caredx (speaking, consulting), Transmedics (consulting), Kamada (consulting), MediGO (consulting), Regeneron (consulting), AstraZeneca (speaking, consulting), Takeda (consulting), and Bridge to Life (speaking).

References

1. Tsipotis, E.; Frey, S.; Connolly, C.; Werbel, W.A.; Chowdhury, R.; Dudley-Brown, S.; Melia, J.M.; Parian, A.M.; Truta, B.; Yu, H.; et al. Antibody response three months after two-dose SARS-CoV-2 mrna vaccination in patients with inflammatory bowel disease. *Am. J. Gastroenterol.* **2022**, *117*, 798–801. [CrossRef] [PubMed]
2. Frey, S.; Chowdhury, R.; Connolly, C.M.; Werbel, W.A.; Segev, D.L.; Parian, A.M.; Tsipotis, E.; Dudley-Brown, S.; Lazarev, M.; Melia, J.M.; et al. Antibody response six months after SARS-CoV-2 mRNA vaccination in patients with inflammatory bowel disease. *Clin. Gastroenterol. Hepatol.* **2022**, *20*, 1609–1612. [CrossRef] [PubMed]
3. Kappelman, M.D.; Weaver, K.N.; Boccieri, M.; Firestine, A.; Zhang, X.; Long, M.D.; Chun, K.; Fernando, M.; Zikry, M.; Dai, X.; et al. Humoral Immune Response to Messenger RNA COVID-19 Vaccines Among Patients with Inflammatory Bowel Disease. *Gastroenterology* **2021**, *161*, 1340–1343.e2. [CrossRef] [PubMed]
4. Kennedy, N.A.; Lin, S.; Goodhand, J.R.; Chanchlani, N.; Hamilton, B.; Bewshea, C.; Nice, R.; Chee, D.; Cummings, J.F.; Fraser, A.; et al. Infliximab is associated with attenuated immunogenicity to BNT162b2 and ChAdOx1 nCoV-19 SARS-CoV-2 vaccines in patients with IBD. *Gut* **2021**, *70*, 1884–1893. [CrossRef] [PubMed]
5. Alexander, J.L.; Kennedy, N.A.; Ibraheim, H.; Anandabaskaran, S.; Saifuddin, A.; Seoane, R.C.; Liu, Z.; Nice, R.; Bewshea, C.; D'Mello, A.; et al. COVID-19 vaccine-induced antibody responses in immunosuppressed patients with inflammatory bowel disease (VIP): A multicentre, prospective, case-control study. *Lancet Gastroenterol. Hepatol.* **2022**, *7*, 342–352. [CrossRef] [PubMed]
6. Edelman-Klapper, H.; Zittan, E.; Shitrit, A.B.-G.; Rabinowitz, K.M.; Goren, I.; Avni-Biron, I.; Ollech, J.E.; Lichtenstein, L.; Banai-Eran, H.; Yanai, H.; et al. Lower serologic response to COVID-19 mrna vaccine in patients with inflammatory bowel diseases treated with anti-tnfα. *Gastroenterology* **2022**, *162*, 454–467. [CrossRef] [PubMed]
7. Planas, D.; Saunders, N.; Maes, P.; Guivel-Benhassine, F.; Planchais, C.; Buchrieser, J.; Bolland, W.H.; Porrot, F.; Staropoli, I.; Lemoine, F.; et al. Considerable escape of SARS-CoV-2 Omicron to antibody neutralization. *Nature* **2022**, *602*, 671–675. [CrossRef] [PubMed]
8. Shenoy, P.; Ahmed, S.; Paul, A.; Cherian, S.; Umesh, R.; Shenoy, V.; Vijayan, A.; Babu, S.; Nivin, S.; Thambi, A. Hybrid immunity versus vaccine-induced immunity against SARS-CoV-2 in patients with autoimmune rheumatic diseases. *Lancet Rheumatol.* **2022**, *4*, e80–e82. [CrossRef] [PubMed]
9. Ahmed, S.; Mehta, P.; Paul, A.; Anu, S.; Cherian, S.; Shenoy, V.; Nalianda, K.K.; Joseph, S.; Poulose, A.; Shenoy, P. Postvaccination antibody titres predict protection against COVID-19 in patients with autoimmune diseases: Survival analysis in a prospective cohort. *Ann. Rheum. Dis.* **2022**, *81*, 868–874. [CrossRef] [PubMed]
10. CDC Center for Disease Control and Prevention [CDC Website]. Interim Clinical Considerations for Use of COVID-19 Vaccines Currently Approved or Authorized in the United States. Available online: https://www.cdc.gov/vaccines/covid-19/clinical-considerations/interim-considerations-us.html#immunocompromised (accessed on 12 May 2022).
11. Pellegrino, R.; Pellino, G.; Selvaggi, L.; Selvaggi, F.; Federico, A.; Romano, M.; Gravina, A.G. BNT162b2 mRNA COVID-19 vaccine is safe in a setting of patients on biologic therapy with inflammatory bowel diseases: A monocentric real-life study. *Expert Rev. Clin. Pharmacol.* **2022**, *15*, 1243–1252. [CrossRef] [PubMed]

12. Li, D.; Debbas, P.; Mujukian, A.; Cheng, S.; Braun, J.; McGovern, D.P.B.; Melmed, G.Y.; CORALE-IBD Study Group. Postvaccination Symptoms After a Third Dose of mRNA SARS-CoV-2 Vaccination in Patients with Inflammatory Bowel Disease: Results from CORALE-IBD. *Inflamm. Bowel Dis.* **2023**, *29*, 883–887. [CrossRef] [PubMed]
13. Galmiche, S.; Nguyen, L.B.L.; Tartour, E.; de Lamballerie, X.; Wittkop, L.; Loubet, P.; Launay, O. Immunological and clinical efficacy of COVID-19 vaccines in immunocompromised populations: A systematic review. *Clin. Microbiol. Infect.* **2022**, *28*, 163–177. [CrossRef] [PubMed]
14. Schell, T.L.; Knutson, K.L.; Saha, S.; Wald, A.; Phan, H.S.; Almasry, M.; Chun, K.; Grimes, I.; Lutz, M.; Hayney, M.S.; et al. Humoral Immunogenicity of 3 COVID-19 Messenger RNA Vaccine Doses in Patients with Inflammatory Bowel Disease. *Inflamm. Bowel Dis.* **2022**, *28*, 1781–1786. [CrossRef] [PubMed]
15. Pavia, G.; Spagnuolo, R.; Quirino, A.; Marascio, N.; Giancotti, A.; Simeone, S.; Cosco, C.; Tino, E.; Carrabetta, F.; Di Gennaro, G.; et al. COVID-19 Vaccine Booster Shot Preserves T Cells Immune Response Based on Interferon-Gamma Release Assay in Inflammatory Bowel Disease (IBD) Patients on Anti-TNFα Treatment. *Vaccines* **2023**, *11*, 591. [CrossRef]
16. Connolly, C.M.; Chiang, T.P.-Y.; Teles, M.; Frey, S.; Alejo, J.L.; Massie, A.; Shah, A.A.; Albayda, J.; Christopher-Stine, L.; Werbel, W.A.; et al. Factors associated with poor antibody response to third-dose SARS-CoV-2 vaccination in patients with rheumatic and musculoskeletal diseases. *Lancet Rheumatol.* **2022**, *4*, e382–e384. [CrossRef]
17. Clarke, K.; Pelton, M.; Stuart, A.; Tinsley, A.; Dalessio, S.; Bernasko, N.; Williams, E.D.; Coates, M. COVID-19 Vaccine Hesitancy in Patients with Inflammatory Bowel Disease. *Dig. Dis. Sci.* **2022**, *67*, 4671–4677. [CrossRef]

Disclaimer/Publisher's Note: The statements, opinions and data contained in all publications are solely those of the individual author(s) and contributor(s) and not of MDPI and/or the editor(s). MDPI and/or the editor(s) disclaim responsibility for any injury to people or property resulting from any ideas, methods, instructions or products referred to in the content.

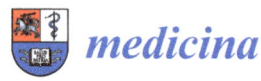

Case Report

Colitis as the Main Presentation of COVID-19: A Case Report

Vlasta Oršić Frič [1,2,*], Vladimir Borzan [1,2], Andrej Borzan [1], Izabela Kiš [3], Branko Dmitrović [1,4] and Ivana Roksandić-Križan [1,5]

1. Faculty of Medicine, Josip Juraj Strossmayer University of Osijek, 31000 Osijek, Croatia
2. Department of Gastroenterology and Hepatology, University Hospital Center Osijek, 31000 Osijek, Croatia
3. Department of Surgery, University Hospital Center Osijek, 31000 Osijek, Croatia
4. Department of Pathology and Forensic Medicine, University Hospital Center Osijek, 31000 Osijek, Croatia
5. Department of Clinical Microbiology and Hospital Infections, University Hospital Center Osijek, 31000 Osijek, Croatia
* Correspondence: vlasta.orsic@gmail.com

Abstract: The main symptoms of coronavirus disease (COVID-19) are fever, cough, tiredness, and loss of smell and taste. Gastrointestinal symptoms are less common. A 38-year-old female patient, previously healthy, presented with a history of hematochezia up to 8 times per day, followed by abdominal cramps, urgency, and chills for two days. She did not have any respiratory symptoms and was previously vaccinated for COVID-19. She was afebrile, with normal vital signs. Blood samples showed normal complete blood count and increased C-reactive protein (CRP), fibrinogen, and D-dimer levels (66 mg/L, 4.1 g/L, and 2302 μ/L FEU, respectively). Stool samples for stool culture, *C. difficile*, and viral examination came back negative. On day 3, she reported a mild cough, fever and loss of smell and taste. Nasopharyngeal swab for SARS-CoV-2 (severe acute respiratory syndrome coronavirus 2) PCR test came back positive. On day 6, the patient still had hematochezia accompanied by abdominal cramps, but fever and respiratory symptoms withdrew. CRP, fibrinogen, and D-dimers were still elevated, as well as liver enzyme levels. Sigmoidoscopy was performed with biopsies taken from sigmoid and rectum for histology and PCR SARS-CoV-2 testing. CT angiography showed no signs of thrombosis in mesenteric veins or arteries. PCR test for SARS-CoV-2 virus from rectal biopsy sample was positive. Patient was treated with methylprednisolone iv for two days and peroral prednisone afterwards, with mesalamine, metronidazole and enoxaparin. Sigmoidoscopy was repeated after two weeks showing only mild hyperemia. At that time, the patient had normal stool, normal CRP, liver enzyme, fibrinogen, and D-dimer levels, and normocytic anemia (hemoglobin level of 103 g/L). We wanted to show that severe gastrointestinal symptoms, such as hemorrhagic colitis, can be the main presentation of COVID-19, even in young patients with no prior comorbidities. In such a case, PCR test in biopsy samples can be performed to prove SARS-CoV-2 infection of bowel mucosa.

Keywords: COVID-19; digestive system infection; gastrointestinal involvement

Citation: Frič, V.O.; Borzan, V.; Borzan, A.; Kiš, I.; Dmitrović, B.; Roksandić-Križan, I. Colitis as the Main Presentation of COVID-19: A Case Report. *Medicina* 2023, *59*, 576. https://doi.org/10.3390/medicina59030576

Academic Editors: Daniel Paramythiotis and Eleni Karlafti

Received: 31 January 2023
Revised: 1 March 2023
Accepted: 10 March 2023
Published: 15 March 2023

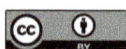

Copyright: © 2023 by the authors. Licensee MDPI, Basel, Switzerland. This article is an open access article distributed under the terms and conditions of the Creative Commons Attribution (CC BY) license (https://creativecommons.org/licenses/by/4.0/).

1. Introduction

In December 2019, novel severe acute respiratory syndrome coronavirus 2 (SARS-CoV-2), which causes coronavirus disease (COVID-19), was identified. The virus rapidly spread around the world causing a global pandemic [1]. The main symptoms of COVID-19 are fever, cough, tiredness, and loss of smell and taste [2]. Gastrointestinal symptoms, such as vomiting and diarrhea, are less common. Here, we present a case of a patient with severe gastrointestinal symptoms as the main clinical presentation of COVID-19.

2. Case Presentation

A 38-year-old female patient, previously healthy, presented with a history of hematochezia up to 8 times per day, followed by abdominal cramps, urgency, and chills for two days. She denied having traveled or having ill contacts, and she did not recall taking any food or medication that could be the cause of her symptoms. She did not have any respiratory symptoms and was previously vaccinated for COVID-19. During physical examination, she was afebrile, with a blood pressure of 110/70 mm Hg, pulse of 60 bpm, and oxygen saturation of 98%, and an abdominal examination showed tenderness in the left lower quadrant of the abdomen. Blood samples showed a normal complete blood count, C-reactive protein (CRP) level of 66 mg/L, fibrinogen level of 4.1 g/L, and D-dimer level of 2302 mcg/L FEU. Stool samples for stool culture, *Clostridioides difficile*, and viral examination were taken, and they came back negative. She received azithromycin 500 mg/day for 3 days and rehydration. On day 3 after the first visit, her CRP levels rose to 89 mg/L, and she reported a mild cough, fever, and loss of smell and taste. A nasopharyngeal swab for SARS-CoV-2 polymerase chain reaction (PCR) test came back positive. On day 6, the patient still had hematochezia accompanied by abdominal cramps, but fever and respiratory symptoms withdrew. CRP level, fibrinogen, and D-dimers were still elevated. Additionally, aspartate aminotransferase (AST) and alanine aminotransferase (ALT) became elevated (78 U/L and 61 U/L, respectively). Gastroenterologist was consulted, and sigmoidoscopy was performed. Sigmoid mucosa showed hyperemia, submucosal bleeding, and erosions (Figure 1); changes were less prominent in rectal mucosa. Biopsies were taken from sigmoid colon and rectum for histology and for PCR SARS-CoV-2 testing (FTD SARS-CoV-2 Assay, Fast Track Diagnostics, Luxembourg). Computed tomography (CT) angiography of mesenteric blood vessels was performed and showed no signs of thrombosis in superior or inferior mesenteric vein or artery, and there was no bowel wall thickening. Histology showed plasma cell and neutrophil infiltration in lamina propria, cryptal abscesses, and cryptal destruction (Figure 2). A PCR test for SARS-CoV-2 virus from colonic biopsy sample was positive. The viral load of the respiratory specimen was higher than that of the rectal specimen, based on the Ct values. The patient was treated with methylprednisolone iv. for two days and peroral prednisone afterwards, with mesalamine orally and rectally, metronidazole orally and enoxaparin. On day 11, the patient was feeling better, with 5–6 normal stools per day with traces of blood; the blood samples showed normal CRP, AST and ALT, fibrinogen 3.7 g/L, and D-dimers 1332 mcg/L FEU. A control sigmoidoscopy was performed two weeks after the first one and showed only mucosal hyperemia (Figure 3). The patient eventually recovered completely with no residual symptoms.

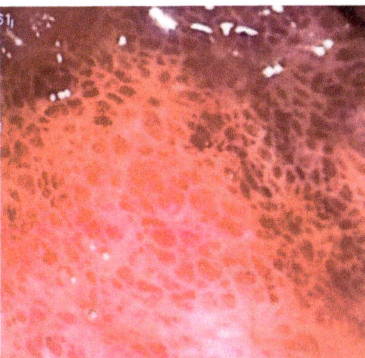

Figure 1. Sigmoidoscopy image of COVID-19 colitis showing submucosal bleeding.

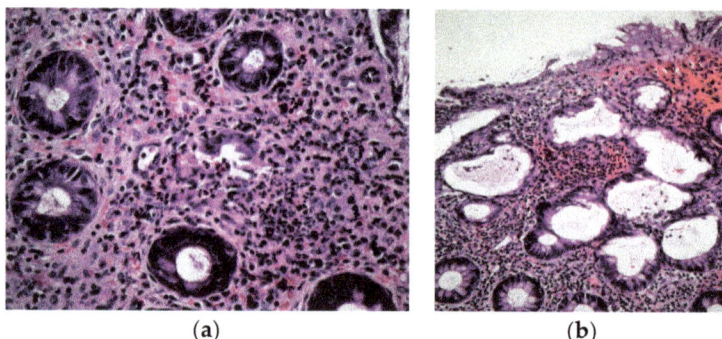

Figure 2. Histology of colonic mucosa: (**a**) Destructed crypt with granulocyte, eosinophil, and plasma cell infiltrate. Hematoxylin and eosin, ×400; (**b**) Neutrophil infiltrate in upper half of lamina propria in colonic mucosa. Hematoxylin and eosin, ×200.

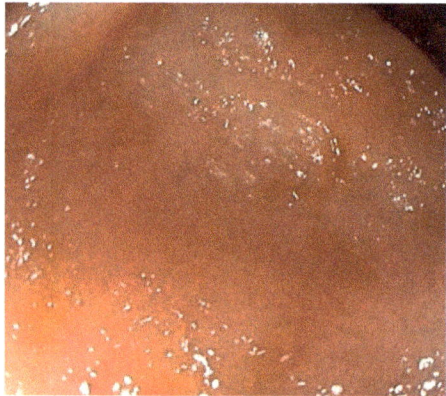

Figure 3. Sigmoidoscopy image of COVID-19 colitis after recovery.

3. Discussion

Our patient presented with a hematochezia, abdominal pain, and chills. As she was previously vaccinated for COVID-19, and she did not have any respiratory symptoms, COVID-19 infection was not suspected at first as the cause of her symptoms. Firstly, infectious colitis due to other possible pathogens was excluded, including bacterial (*Salmonella* spp., *Shigella* spp., *Escherichia coli*, *Yersinia enterocolitica*, *Campylobacter jejuni*), viral (Norovirus, Adenovirus) and *C. difficile* infection (glutamate dehydrogenase antigen toxin screen). It is now well known that SARS-CoV-2 infection can cause gastrointestinal symptoms in 12% up to more than 60% of patients [3,4], and, in some, they can even precede or be present without respiratory symptoms [5]. Most common gastrointestinal symptoms of COVID-19 are diarrhea, nausea, and vomiting [6], and symptoms of hemorrhagic colitis were reported only in several cases so far [7,8].

SARS-CoV-2 binds to angiotensin-converting enzyme (ACE) 2, which is expressed in the gastrointestinal epithelial cells, among other tissues. Viral nucleocapside protein and viral RNA were also detected in gastrointestinal epithelial cells, proving that SARS-CoV-2 could cause gastrointestinal infection [9]. Qian et al. [10] found coronavirus virions in rectal tissue observed under the electron microscopy, also proving that SARS-CoV-2 can cause active gastrointestinal infection. Furthermore, SARS-CoV-2 RNA was detected in stool samples in around half of the patients [9] with COVID-19. Unfortunately, viral stool sampling was performed only for Norovirus and Adenovirus, and SARS-CoV-2 virus was not determined in stool samples of this patient. From data published so far, it is known that SARS-CoV-2 can cause ischemic colitis in patients with severe COVID-19 infection, due to hemodynamic instability and vasopressor therapy. That was not the case in our patient, who was young, with no comorbidities, with a mild course of COVID-19, and without hemodynamic instability. COVID-19 infection itself could cause coagulopathy in large and small blood vessels by causing endotheliitis and systemic inflammation [11,12], leading to various thrombotic vascular conditions, ischemic colitis being among them. An international multicenter study of COVID-19 patients undergoing endoscopy showed that around third of the patients had changes that resemble ischemic colopathy [13].

Differential diagnosis of acute, hemorrhagic colitis is diverse. Besides infectious agents, acute colitis can be caused by inflammatory bowel disease, ischemia, drugs, neutropenia, radiation, etc. [14].

Considering the age of the patient, the first manifestation of ulcerative colitis could be considered as a cause of her symptoms. Ulcerative colitis is an inflammatory bowel disease in which inflammation involves rectal mucosa, but it can also extend to more proximal parts of the large bowel. Most common symptoms of ulcerative colitis are diarrhea, rectal bleeding, tenesmus, and urgency. During endoscopy, changes seen can be mild, such as mucosal hyperemia or decreased vascular pattern, to more pronounced, such as erosions, ulcerations, or spontaneous bleeding. Changes spread continuously from rectum to more proximal parts of the colon. In this patient, endoscopic findings did not correspond completely to findings that can usually be seen in patients with ulcerative colitis. For example, rectal mucosa was almost normal [15].

Another inflammatory bowel disease that can be the cause of colitis and hematochezia is Crohn's disease of the colon. Most common symptoms of Crohn's disease are diarrhea and abdominal pain, but fever, fatigue, anemia, and other systemic symptoms can also appear. Endoscopic findings in Crohn's colitis are aphthous ulcers or presence of deep ulcers that cause cobblestone appearance of the colonic mucosa. Rectum is usually spared. On abdominal CT scan in Crohn's disease patients, discontinuous lesions can be seen, as well as bowel wall thickening reflecting the transmural nature of the inflammation [16].

Besides the SARS-CoV-2 virus, ischemic colitis can also be caused by thrombotic or embolic events within large mesenteric arteries, drugs, vasculitis, volvulus, strenuous physical activity, shock, etc. It usually affects the population older than 65 years of age, with cardiovascular comorbidities or diabetes mellitus. In younger patients, ischemic colitis is usually caused by various drugs (such as oral contraceptives, nasal decongestants, and cocaine), vasculitis, coagulation disorders, or heavy exercise. Colon is especially susceptible to ischemia due to its relatively low blood flow and its sensitivity to autonomic stimulation. The most common symptoms of ischemic colitis are hematochezia, diarrhea, abdominal pain, and urgency, and it is usually characterized with an abrupt onset of symptoms. Abdominal CT imaging and colonoscopy are diagnostic methods of choice. CT imaging shows bowel wall thickening, bowel dilation, and thumbprinting. Pneumatosis or portal vein gas can also be seen in severe cases. During colonoscopy, segmental distribution and rectal sparing are common. Hyperemia, with or without ulceration, and submucosal hemorrhage are usually found. Biopsies should be obtained, and typical findings are mucosal and submucosal oedema and hemorrhage, with erythrocyte extravasation in lamina propria [14,17].

Colitis caused by drugs can be manifested as a drug reaction with eosinophilia and systemic symptoms (DRESS) syndrome, which is characterized not only by fever, eosinophilia, skin rash, and lymphadenopathy, but also by visceral organ involvement, such as colitis. It can be caused by various drugs, but most commonly by karbamazepine. The main symptoms of DRESS colitis are diarrhea (with or without hematochezia) and abdominal pain, and symptoms usually appear weeks after exposure to the culprit drug. The course of DRESS syndrome is usually unpredictable, and delayed autoimmune sequelae can develop. During colonoscopy, ulcerations can sometimes be found. On histology, eosinophil and plasma cell infiltration is typically seen [18].

In this case, the most probable cause of the patient's symptoms was SARS-CoV-2 infection. SARS-CoV-2 PCR tests, both in the nasopharyngeal swab and sigmoid biopsy sample, came back positive. The patient had fever and other respiratory symptoms of COVID-19, although they were mild and short term. Moreover, elevated liver transaminase levels and D-dimers also pointed to the viral cause of her symptoms. Other possible infective causes were excluded. Clinical symptoms, with the abrupt appearance of hematochezia and abdominal pain, and no prior history of gastrointestinal symptoms did not point in favor of inflammatory bowel disease, and neither did endoscopy findings. Additionally, the patient recovered completely and did not have any more disease flares, even though she was not taking any medication to maintain the disease remission. Ischemia due to thromboembolic incidents of large mesenteric arteries or veins was excluded by CT angiography and was not probable, as the patient was young and without comorbidities. Other potential causes of ischemic colitis, besides SARS-CoV-2 infection, were also excluded. Lastly, colitis caused by drugs, such as the one that appears as a part of DRESS syndrome, was not likely, as the patient denied taking any drugs prior to beginning of her symptoms. Therefore, in our patient, hemorrhagic colitis was caused either by direct cytopathic effect of viral infection in colonic mucosa or by focal ischemic changes due to coagulopathy in small blood vessels of the colon. Our finding that viral load from nasopharyngeal swab was higher than from colonic biopsy samples, was consistent with previous reports that viral loads from respiratory tract samples are usually much higher than in non-respiratory samples. High viral loads from samples from upper respiratory tract are not related with clinical manifestations and can also be found in asymptomatic patients. This can be explained by the fact that higher viral load poses a greater risk for further transmission of the virus [19]. The lower viral load in bowel mucosa in this patient shows that probably both the cytopathic effect of viral replication in epithelial cells of bowel mucosa and focal ischemia due to coagulopathy were the cause of hemorrhagic colitis.

As no conclusive data on the treatment of hemorrhagic colitis which accompanies COVID-19 was published at the time of this case, therapy was given to address potential causes and consequences of inflammatory changes in bowel mucosa. As it was suspected that both viral infection of colonic mucosa and coagulopathy of colonic small blood vessels were cause of symptoms in our patient, she was treated with corticosteroids to lower the inflammatory burden of COVID-19 infection systemically. Mesalamine is a medication used in ulcerative colitis as a systemic and topical treatment. It is shown that it reduces inflammation of the intestinal mucosa acting locally. It is a safe and well-tolerated medication, with proven efficacy in mild to moderate ulcerative colitis [20]. In this patient, we used mesalamine to lower the inflammatory burden locally in the intestinal mucosa. Small-dose low-molecular-weight heparin (LMWH) was given to address the possible coagulopathy. Metronidazole was firstly used ex juvantibus, to address the possible *C. difficile* infection. When the result came back negative, it was continued to lower the possibility of bacterial translocation from bowel lumen to bloodstream.

4. Conclusions

Data about COVID-19 colitis are scarce. We wanted to show that severe gastrointestinal symptoms, such as hemorrhagic colitis, can be the main presentation of COVID-19, even in young patients with no prior comorbidities. In such a case, a PCR test in biopsy samples can be performed to prove SARS-CoV-2 infection of bowel mucosa. Combination of corticosteroid therapy, mesalamine and LMWH showed to be effective in our patient.

Author Contributions: V.O.F., V.B. and A.B. collected data for manuscript preparation. V.O.F. and I.K. wrote the manuscript draft. B.D. prepared histology reports and images. I.R.-K. prepared microbiology reports. V.B., I.R.-K. and B.D. undertook critical revision of the manuscript. All authors have read and agreed to the published version of the manuscript.

Funding: This research received no external funding.

Institutional Review Board Statement: Not applicable.

Informed Consent Statement: Written informed consent has been obtained from the patient to publish this paper.

Data Availability Statement: All data regarding the findings are available within the manuscript.

Conflicts of Interest: The authors declare no conflict of interest.

References

1. World Health Organization. Situation Report-51 Situation in Numbers Total and New Cases in Last 24 Hours. Available online: https://apps.who.int/iris/handle/10665/331475 (accessed on 29 July 2022).
2. Long, B.; Carius, B.M.; Liang, S.Y.; Chavez, S.; Brady, W.J.; Koyfman, A.; Gottlieb, M. Clinical update on COVID-19 for the emergency clinician: Presentation and evaluation. *Am. J. Emerg. Med.* **2022**, *54*, 46–57. [CrossRef] [PubMed]
3. Parasa, S.; Desai, M.; Chandrasekar, V.T.; Patel, H.K.; Kennedy, K.F.; Roesch, T.; Sharma, P. Prevalence of Gastrointestinal Symptoms and Fecal Viral Shedding in Patients With Coronavirus Disease 2019: A Systematic Review and Meta-analysis. *JAMA Netw Open* **2020**, *3*, e2011335. [CrossRef] [PubMed]
4. Redd, W.D.; Zhou, J.C.; Hathorn, K.E.; McCarty, T.R.; Bazarbashi, A.N.; Thompson, C.C.; Chan, W.W. Prevalence and Characteristics of Gastrointestinal Symptoms in Patients With Severe Acute Respiratory Syndrome Coronavirus 2 Infection in the United States: A Multicenter Cohort Study. *Gastroenterology* **2020**, *159*, 765–767.e2. [CrossRef] [PubMed]
5. Pan, L.; Mu, M.I.; Yang, P.; Sun, Y.; Wang, R.; Yan, J.; Tu, L. Clinical characteristics of COVID-19 patients with digestive symptoms in Hubei, China: A descriptive, cross-sectional, multicenter study. *Am. J. Gastroenterol.* **2020**, *115*, 766–773. [CrossRef] [PubMed]
6. Cao, T.T.; Zhang, G.Q.; Pellegrini, E.; Zhao, Q.; Li, J.; Luo, L.J.; Pan, H.Q. COVID-19 and its effects on the digestive system. *World J. Gastroenterol.* **2021**, *27*, 3502–3515. [CrossRef] [PubMed]
7. Carvalho, A.; Alqusairi, R.; Adams, A.; Paul, M.; Kothari, N.; Peters, S.; DeBenedet, A.T. SARS-CoV-2 Gastrointestinal Infection Causing Hemorrhagic Colitis: Implications for Detection and Transmission of COVID-19 Disease. *Am. J. Gastroenterol.* **2020**, *115*, 942–946. [CrossRef] [PubMed]
8. Uhlenhopp, D.J.; Ramachandran, R.; Then, E.; Parvataneni, S.; Grantham, T.; Gaduputi, V. COVID-19-Associated Ischemic Colitis: A Rare Manifestation of COVID-19 Infection—Case Report and Review. *J. Investig. Med. High Impact. Case Rep.* **2022**, *10*, 23247096211065625. [CrossRef] [PubMed]
9. Xiao, F.; Tang, M.; Zheng, X.; Liu, Y.; Li, X.; Shan, H. Evidence for Gastrointestinal Infection of SARS-CoV-2. *Gastroenterology* **2020**, *158*, 1831–1833.e3. [CrossRef] [PubMed]
10. Qian, Q.; Fan, L.; Liu, W.; Li, J.; Yue, J.; Wang, M.; Jiang, C. Direct Evidence of Active SARS-CoV-2 Replication in the Intestine. *Clin. Infect. Dis.* **2021**, *73*, 361–366. [CrossRef] [PubMed]
11. Levi, M.; Thachil, J.; Iba, T.; Levy, J.H. Coagulation abnormalities and thrombosis in patients with COVID-19. *Lancet Haematol.* **2020**, *7*, e438–40. [CrossRef] [PubMed]
12. Varga, Z.; Flammer, A.J.; Steiger, P.; Haberecker, M.; Andermatt, R.; Zinkernagel, A.S.; Moch, H. Endothelial cell infection and endotheliitis in COVID-19. *Lancet* **2020**, *395*, 1417–1418. [CrossRef] [PubMed]
13. Vanella, G.; Capurso, G.; Burti, C.; Fanti, L.; Ricciardiello, L.; Lino, A.S.; Arcidiacono, P.G. Gastrointestinal mucosal damage in patients with COVID-19 undergoing endoscopy: An international multicentre study. *BMJ Open Gastroenterol.* **2021**, *8*, e000578. [CrossRef] [PubMed]
14. Abreu, M.T.; Harpaz, N. Diagnosis of colitis: Making the initial diagnosis. *Clin. Gastroenterol. Hepatol.* **2007**, *5*, 295–301. [CrossRef] [PubMed]
15. Kobayashi, T.; Siegmund, B.; Le Berre, C.; Wei, S.C.; Ferrante, M.; Shen, B.; Bernstein, C.N.; Danese, S.; Peyrin-Biroulet, L.; Hibi, T. Ulcerative colitis. *Nat. Rev. Dis. Prim.* **2020**, *6*, 74. [CrossRef] [PubMed]
16. Roda, G.; Ng, S.C.; Kotze, P.G.; Argollo, M.; Panaccione, R.; Spinelli, A.; Kaser, A.; Peyrin-Biroulet, L.; Danese, S. Crohn's disease. *Nat. Rev. Dis. Prim.* **2020**, *6*, 22. [CrossRef] [PubMed]
17. Xu, Y.; Xiong, L.; Li, Y.; Jiang, X.; Xiong, Z. Diagnostic methods and drug therapies in patients with ischemic colitis. *Int. J. Color. Dis.* **2021**, *36*, 47–56. [CrossRef] [PubMed]
18. Jevtic, D.; Dumic, I.; Nordin, T.; Singh, A.; Sulovic, N.; Radovanovic, M.; Milovanovic, T. Less Known Gastrointestinal Manifestations of Drug Reaction with Eosinophilia and Systemic Symptoms (DRESS) Syndrome: A Systematic Review of the Literature. *J. Clin. Med.* **2021**, *10*, 4287. [CrossRef] [PubMed]
19. Puhach, O.; Meyer, B.; Eckerle, I. SARS-CoV-2 viral load and shedding kinetics. *Nat. Rev. Microbiol.* **2023**, *21*, 147–161. [CrossRef]
20. Paridaens, K.; Fullarton, J.R.; Travis, S.P.L. Efficacy and safety of oral Pentasa (prolonged-release mesalazine) in mild-to-moderate ulcerative colitis: A systematic review and meta-analysis. *Curr. Med. Res. Opin.* **2021**, *37*, 1891–1900. [CrossRef] [PubMed]

Disclaimer/Publisher's Note: The statements, opinions and data contained in all publications are solely those of the individual author(s) and contributor(s) and not of MDPI and/or the editor(s). MDPI and/or the editor(s) disclaim responsibility for any injury to people or property resulting from any ideas, methods, instructions or products referred to in the content.

MDPI
St. Alban-Anlage 66
4052 Basel
Switzerland
www.mdpi.com

Medicina Editorial Office
E-mail: medicina@mdpi.com
www.mdpi.com/journal/medicina

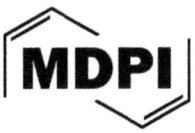

Disclaimer/Publisher's Note: The statements, opinions and data contained in all publications are solely those of the individual author(s) and contributor(s) and not of MDPI and/or the editor(s). MDPI and/or the editor(s) disclaim responsibility for any injury to people or property resulting from any ideas, methods, instructions or products referred to in the content.

www.ingramcontent.com/pod-product-compliance
Lightning Source LLC
LaVergne TN
LVHW070601100526
838202LV00012B/534